D1881160

HEALTH AWARENESS FOR WOMEN

HEALTH AWARENESS FOR WOMEN

Edited by
Dr. Vatsala Samant (M.D. Bom.)

GYAN PUBLISHING HOUSE
NEW DELHI - 110002

HEALTH AWARENESS FOR WOMEN

(Health)

© Dr. Vatsala Samant (M.D. Bom.)

ISBN : 9788121206464

All rights are reserved. No part of this book may be reproduced in any manner without written permission.

Published in 2000 in India by
Gyan Publishing House
5, Ansari Road
New Delhi 110 002
Laser Typesetting: Grow Computers, Delhi
Printed at: Mehra Offset Press, New Delhi

DEDICATED
TO
WOMEN OF ALLAHABAD
BY
THE WOMEN DOCTORS
OF ALLAHABAD

CONTENTS

	Foreword	11
	Preface	13
	Acknowledgements	17
	List of Contributors	19
1.	Anatomy of Reproductive System: Internal Organs	21
2.	Menstruation	27
3.	Menopause	31
4.	Breast	35
5.	Conception	39
6.	Development of the Embryo	43
7.	Pregnancy	47
8.	Problems During Pregnancy	51
9.	Abortion	53
10.	Child Birth—Labour	55
11.	RCH—Reproductive Child Health	61
12.	Hazards of Puerperium and Post-Natal Period	63
13.	Toll of Maternity	65
14.	Family Planning	67
15.	Contraception	69
16.	Infertility	75
17.	Care of the Newborn Baby	83
18.	Immunization	85
19.	Premature Babies	87
20.	Breast Feeding	89
21.	Fever in Children	93

22. Gastroenteritis in Children 95
23. Some Childhood Deformities 97
24. Congenital Malfomations 101
25. Dyslexia 105
26. Ageing 107
27. Glaucoma 111
28. Cataract 113
29. Varicose Veins 117
30. Rheumatoid Arthritis 119
31. Osteoarthritis 121
32. Osteoporosis 123
33. Staying Healthy the Natural Way 127
34. Pregnancy and Its Hazards 131
35. Operative Procedures in Obstetries and Gynaecology 135
36. Ultrasound 139
37. Maternal Mortality 141
38. Genital Hygiene 143
39. Vaginal Discharge 145
40. Urinary Track Disturbance 147
41. Infection 149
42. Leukoplakia 153
43. Cancer of the Reproductive System 155
44. Cancer of the Reproductive Organs 159
45. Role of Radiotherapy in the Treatment of Cancer 165
46. Breast Cancer 171
47. Defence Systmes of the Body 175
48. AIDS 179
49. Sex Education 183
50. Hormones 187
51. Thyroid 189
52. Fitness 193

53. Aerobics 203
54. Exercise and Diet 205
55. Yoga 211
56. Physiotherapy 217
57. Acupuncture 219
58. Backache 221
59. Intersex 223
60. Hysteria 225
61. Diabetes 227
62. Fibromyalgia 238
63. Malaria 241
64. Anaemia 243
65. Tuberculosis 247
66. Hepatitis B 251
67. Obesity 253
68. Sleep: A Divine Gift 255
69. Counselling: A Therapy 259
70. Pathology 263
71. Infectious Viral Diseases 267
72. Endoscopy 273
73. Massage 279
74. Homeopathy 281
75. Water or Hydrotherapy 283
76. Ayurveda's Therapy or Medicine 285
77. Science of Relaxation 287
78. Tips for Meditation and also Relaxations 289
79. Epilogue 291
Index 293

FOREWORD

Born on 19th January, 1910 at Bassein, Bombay, Dr. (Mrs.) Vatsala Samant Chowdhry had her early education at Bombay. She joined the Salt Satyagraha in 1929-30 and was jailed. She obtained MBBS and MD degrees in 1936 and 1938, respectively from the Bombay University. A recipient of Dr. Shirvalkar, Gold Medal in Surgery, she was also awarded the Prince of Wales Gold Medal and the Hansraj Pragji Fellowship of the Bombay University in MD examination.

After working as Assistant Honorary Obstetrician Gynaecologist at Cama Aldless Hospital for some time, she joined the Kamla Nehru Memorial Hospital, Allahabad in 1942 as the Medical Superintendent. She has been the Professor and Head of Department of Obstetrics and Gynaecology at the Motilal Nehru Medical College, Allahabad since 1963 and the Chief Investigator of Indian Council of Medical Research Work at Kamla Nehru Memorial Hospital, since 1967. She visited America under Leaders Programme in 1951 and is President of Association of Obstetrics and Gynaecology, Allahabad Branch.

She has presented papers at various national and international conferences and has a number of publications to her credit.

She was awarded Padma Shri in 1972. She was a member of the National Committee for Celebration of 40th Anniversary of Independence and Jawaharlal Nehru Centenary.

The residents of Allahabad take the name of Dr. V. Samant with great pride and affection because she has been and is a leading Gynaecologist of the city and has worked for the welfare of the masses with compassion and complete dedication.

After completing her glorious term as Superintendent of Kamla Nehru Memorial Hospital, Dr. Samant joined Nazareth Hospital in 1975. She looked after and established the Department of Obstetrics and Gynaecology and rendered valuable service for nineteen long years.

Even at her age when most people retire she is still active professionally and is engaged in writing a book to make common people aware about some common medical Obstetrical and Gynaecological problems. Indeed her commitment to work is a source of inspiration for the younger generation.

Dr. (Mrs.) Navneeta Banerjee
Sr. Consultant (Gynaecologist)
Kamla Nehru Memorial Hospital
Allahabad.

PREFACE

I have been practising as a specialist in women's diseases and thus I had an opportunity to come across thousands of women, rich and poor, belonging to various castes and creeds, I have noticed that our women particularly from middle class and rural areas neglect themselves as far as their health is concerned. They are busy doing domestic chores, looking after the welfare of the family, husband, children essential till they become seriously ill.

While performing the vital function of motherhood they pay the price either in permanent disability or even in death. Maternal mortality or death rate is very high in India and so also the infant death rate. To deliver a healthy baby and remain healthy is a must for a woman. She is the one who is responsible for producing healthy generation and to ensure this, it is quite necessary to teach her about health awareness. Teach a woman and you teach a family.

An idea of writing a book on health for women was there right from the beginning of my medical superintendantship at Kamala Nehru Hospital. But due to workload, illness, domestic problems, I was unable to put them on paper.

After my retirement from Nazreth Hospital in 1995, the seed of writing was sown. Not being a writer, it took me some time to sit down and put on paper my ideas about health awareness. A small book was ready after some research.

My idea of writing this book, which is easy to read and understand, is to teach women the basic facts about regarding normal functions of reproduction and health care. Nothing is more important than our health, to enjoy our life. The aim of this book, as I have said is to spell out facts of life we need to know, and a package of knowledge for making our women fitter and healthier in mind and body.

To ease my burden and in order to encourage my pupils and younger gynaecologists I requested some of my juniors to write chapters on the subjects they are practising and they agreed to do so. Thus it is the work of the oldest and young gynaecologists of Allahabad—a booklet explaining the natural facts of life and diseases, easy to read and understand. I hope it will benefit our womenfolk. I have purposely avoided treatment as I believe a doctor has to decide the treatment and not the patient.

What is gynaecology? It is a word derived from Greek. Meaning *gyn*—women, and *logy* meaning discussion regarding a woman or study of women.

When a woman seeks advice for discomfort related to Genital organs we must think that her need is of understanding a whole woman as such, her outlook, her achievement, failures, and her domestic and social problems, and thus a gynaecologist should also be a psychologist.

When one is young one never thinks of growing old and pays no mind to age. Youth lies to us, blinds us, gives us a false sense of immortality, makes us believe, we are supreme, unbeatable and everlasting. How frightening it is to learn that we are only too mortal vulnerable and that in the end we have to die.

I used to feel so strong, so vigorous, so full of zest. But lately I have started feeling worn out. It is as if all the life has been drained out of me.

Life lived to the fullest. When we grow old, things happen to destroy the fabric of our existence, age makes it easier to cope in so many ways. We have acquired an understanding, wisdom is ours and we have life's experience to draw on and sustain us.

Whereas in our youth troubles come to plague us, we have few weapons with which to combat them, no ready references, no old knowledge stored in us, no inner resources to see us through. They overwhelm and can destroy us.

Life is hard. It is meant to be hard. To test us, to test our mettle, it breaks us or makes us. And the lessons of life are equally hard, yet if we are astute and quick, then we only have to learn these lessons once.

What, must happen will happen. Nothing can stop it.

I having gone through many ailments of ageing. I thought it will be worthwhile to create awareness amongst all members of our society including the young and old about ailments that can come before them.

Even if one woman in ten benefits by reading this book on health awareness one I shall be happy have my dream come true.

What I am today is due the women of Allahabad who had trust in me regarding ailments and nothing acts to a doctor more than the trust or confidence in you which is just like a shot of adranalin worth a million dollars.

I thought it would be in the fitness of thing to dedicate this book to women of Allahabad and so this book is a culmination of a long desire which had begun long ago.

I have been able to bring my dream of writing into form through the kind cooperation of Gyan Publishing House who have shown great interest in bringing this book out in such a short time.

Dr. Vatsala Samant

ACKNOWLEDGEMENTS

Assistance and encouragement showered on me by my co-writers, patients, friends, my near and dear ones I mean the family members has been over-whelming and I thank them all. Among them I must name Mrs Beena Nair, Principal of a school, a patient whom I have gifted with two sons but more than that a good friend of mine. She offered herself to edit my manuscript, we used to have lunch sessions and start editing and end in the evening with a little gossip. She knowing my age being vulnerable, used to goad me to finish the work. I thank her for her companionship, her friendly rapport and her sister-in-law Nillu for serving delicious lunches.

Mr Naresh Agarwal and his wife Ujwala who helped me to computerise the manuscript in their printing press.

Dr Navneeta Banerjee who willingly wrote a foreword to my book. My co-writers who obliged me by writing articles that are included in the book.

Dr Mitali Tandon PhD., mother of my grand daughter-in-law, I approached her at the last moment and she immediately obliged me by writing an article on councelling. My publishers who agreed to publish the book despite the fact that this is the first book they are publishing on health awareness and written by a person for the first time and unknown in the literary world.

Dr. Vandana Bansal D.G.O. Incharge of Geeta Jyoti Hospital in Allahabad. I am grateful to you fro writing an article on Endoscopy.

I thank them all.

Last but not least my near and dear ones.

My daughter Mrs Sasmeeta Srivastava for doing final computerisation for providing literature for consultation.

My nephew, Anil Chowdhry IPS for taking me to the publishers to telephoning them as I am hard of hearing, getting me books to consulted discussing the subjects and giving me moral support and his wife's hospitality during my stay with her.

My grandchildren who helped in typing, etc.

Had it not been for the help and encouragement that I got this book would not have seen the light of the day.

LIST OF CONTRIBUTORS

1. **Dr. Manjula Pande** (M.S.)	Head of the Deptt. of Obstetrical and Gynaecologist at Nazareth Hospital, Allahabad
2. **Dr. Manju Varma** (M.S.)	Professor of Obstetrical and Gynaecologist at Motilal Nehru Medical College, Allahabad
3. **Dr. Sarita Bajaj**	PhD., Professor Motilal Nehru Medical College, Allahabad
4. **Dr. Abhilasha Chaturvedi**	D.G.O. Incharge of IVF Center at Allahabad
5. **Dr. Madhavi Mital**	M.D. U.S.G. expert, Incharge of Ultrasound and Mamography Center
6. **Dr. Radharani Dutt Chaudhary (Ghosh)**	M.S.D.M. Radiologist Begum Azad Wing, Kamla Nehru Hospital, Allahabad
7. **Dr. Abha Mallick**	MD Practicing Paedetrician, Allahabad
8. **Dr. Mitali Tandon**	MSW - TISS, PhD. - Annasalai - Practicing Counsellor
9. **Dr. Nivedita Banerjee**	M.D. Prof., Kamla Nehru Hospital, Allahabad.
10. **Dr. Vandana Bansal**	M.B.B.S. D.G.U. Incharge of Jeevan Jyoti Hospital, Allahabad

1

ANATOMY OF REPRODUCTIVE SYSTEM: INTERNAL ORGANS

Dr. Vatsala Samant

Ovaries

Ovaries are female sexual glands. They store millions of eggs but only one egg comes out on the surface and if not fertilized by the sperm of male sexual gland, the egg perishes and there is bleeding from the uterus. This happens every month and is known as menstruation. There is another very important function performed by the ovaries that is production of female hormones. These hormones are responsible for development of secondary sexual characteristics and development of genital system, that is, transformation of a girl into an adult woman.

There are two ovaries on right and left side of the uterus as shown in Fig. 1.

Fallopian Tubes

These are two in number left and right on either side of the uterus and as shown in the figure they connect ovaries to the uterus to allow passage of the sperm from the uterus to the ovary and fertilized ovum from these to the uterus. They are thin walled and incapable to develop the ovum but if blocked by infection hinder fertility.

Uterus

It is a muscular organ situated in the lower abdomen in the centre as shown in the figure. It is lined by a coating and has three openings—two at the top and one down below which opens in the vagina. The lower part of the uterus with the opening is known as

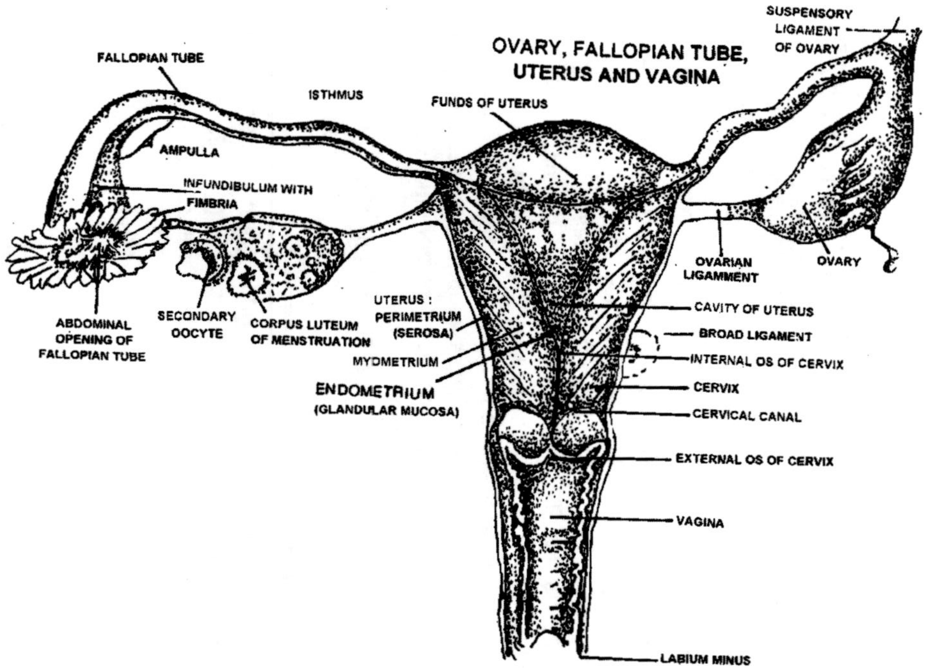

Fig. 1 : Anatomy of Reproductive System: Internal Organs.

neck or cervix. The function of the uterus is to embed the fertilized ovum, to nourish it and protect if from heat and cold for nine months.

Vagina

A muscular open space which connects the cervical opening with the outside and is closed by the cribriform membrane known as hymen which is torn during coitus.

External Organs

There are two lips which protect the vaginal opening. These are known as *Labia minora* and *Labia majora* which are on the right and left side. There is also a *clitoris* which is a small highly sensitive organ located in front of the opening of the vagina. The *Urethra* is the opening of the urinary bladder which is above the vaginal opening. Below the vaginal opening is the anus for defecation.

Puberty

Puberty is the onset of sexual maturity in humans when the secondary sexual characteristics appear and the reproductive organs become functional.

It is attainment of womanhood. A girl developes into a full-fledged woman ready to procreate. The age at which this transformation happens varies from country to country. It depends on the climate, family background and play of hormones. Physical changes take place. Breasts represented by tiny nipples on the chest start growing. Hair starts growing on the pubic and axilla. She starts her menstrual period.

The period between puberty and adolescence is a period of stress and strain not only physical but also emotional. This is a period of life during which a carefree child becomes a responsible adult. She is interested in her appearance, becomes moody, secretive, imaginative and curious. It takes a little time to achieve physical and emotional maturity and thus the management during this period becomes difficult.

The girl should not be teased and her move towards independence should be respected, sometimes to be controlled within limits.

Affection and trust should take place of orders. She should be encouraged to be occupied in work, a healthy recreation within the limits of physical strength. Even before the onset of puberty, the mother can make the girl aware about menstruation and clear her doubts about the changes taking place in her body.

It is a well-known fact that after attaining puberty, very often the periods are irregular, scanty, painful but there is nothing to worry about this phenomena. In due course of time, periods become regular though the pain during menses continues. Some girls have bouts of vomiting, fever and malaise. A pill of analgesie or Antispasmodic medicine such as Spasmodon is helpful in allaying the pain. There are a few instances where a girl does not attain puberty. She should be investigated. Hormonal imbalance, congenital anomalies, chronic diseases like Tuberculosis, Anaemia are some of the causes of non-attainment of puberty.

Delayed Puberty

The lack of onset of pubertal characteristics—breast or pubic hair growth by age 13 and the lack of menarche by age 15 represents a significant delay. Also lack of pubertal development by 4 years after onset suggests the need for evaluation for possible hormone deficiency, causes hypergonadotropic or hypogonadotropic genetic etiology, ovarian failure or it may be due to ingoing physical, emotional or systematic conditions. These should not be treated with HRT cyclic oestrogens and progestron. If menses are delayed after the age of 16 years the doctor should be consulted.

Precocious or Early Puberty

Secondary sexual characteristics such as enlargement of the breasts occurring in a girl before the age of 8 years is known as precocious puberty. It is a manifestation of a tumour of the ovary and brain syndrome. A case has been quoted from Lima Madena in Peru where not only did the child have an early onset of puberty and menses but delivered a baby at the age of 5 years and 9 months. She was suffering from syndrome of the brain.

Precocious puberty is a disorder characterized by partial or complete change occurring in girls less than 7 years of age and in boys less than 9 years of age. In true precocious puberty menstruation is isosexual and complete and is mediated by the antiriar pituitary gland and therefore it is appropriate for the sex of child. In contrast, pseudo precocious puberty is not mediated by pituitary hormones and is typically incomplete and is either heterosexual or isosexual. A boy presenting this condition may be due to brain tumour causing it than in the case of a girl, but precocious puberty is more common in girls.

I know of a case in which a girl aged 5 years belonging to Banda district had all the evidence of early onset of puberty. Her breasts were developed and also other secondary sexual characteristics and she was menstruating. Rumour floated in the district that a Devi or Goddess was born and people started worshipping and bestowed gifts. Parents were displaying her and earning money. I happened to know the District Magistrate and requested him to send the girl to Kamla Nehru Hospital. X-ray of the abdomen showed it to be a case of Malignant Feminising Tumour of the ovary. We requested the parents that she can be cured by surgery and the symptoms would disappear but unfortunately operation was refused and I am sure the girl must have died due to cancer of the ovary, an example of sheer ignorance.

PMS Syndrome

PMS or premenstrual syndrome is a symptom complex which precedes onset of menstrual bleeding and the symptoms are headache, insomnia, back pain, abdominal cramps, mental confusion and emotional upset, mild breast tenderness, fluid retention, bloated feeling, anxiety, dietary, cravings, irritability and inability to concentrate. PMS is terrible. Unfortunately neither the cause nor the cure for PMS is currently known. However the following measures may help alleviate some of the symptoms: A balanced diet—grains, fruits, vegetables and moderate amount of meat and milk products must be taken. Exercise regularly to reduce stress and keep the body fit.

It has also been shown to be effective in the treatment of depression. The person should avoid alcohol and coffee, reduce excessive salt in the diet to reduce fluid retention. If you experience low blood sugar such as fatigue, dizziness, divide the meals into six mini meals rich in carbohydrates and protein and low in simple sugars. B-complex vitamins, calcium and pain relieving medicines help to some extent. Walking is often one of the best thing to relieve it.

2

MENSTRUATION

Dr. Vatsala Samant

Menses or menstruation is a periodic and cyclical shedding of the membrane of the uterus or womb accompanied by loss of blood. It occurs approximately at 28 days cycle between puberty and menopause. It is a function peculiar to women.

The uterus is under the control of ovarian secretion or hormones and prepares itself to lodge a fertilized ovum. If conception or pregnancy does not happen, shedding and bleeding from the uterus takes place. First period may be short or long and cycle irregular. Regular rhythm is usually established within two to three years. Some girls may not have periods for 2-12 months. Each woman has her own rhythm which may change after marriage and child bearing. Any cycle between three to five weeks is supposed to be normal. Similarly there is a wide variation in the duration and amount of blood loss. Three to five days duration or even two to seven days is normal. Menses has been a subject of taboo and superstition, and folklore is responsible for causing abnormal reactions in young girls. It was known as an unclean period which instils feelings of shame, embarassment and resentment. Mothers teach their daughters that they are in low physical state and vulnerable to all manner of ills and so should not take bath during these days, they were isolated and treated as untouchables. This is a wrong attitude and now it has been changed. The girls should be explained simply and truthfully that it is a manifestation of womanhood. They should live their normal life, play and bathe, etc.

General Disturbance Associated with Menses

Most of the women suffer minor physical and nervous disturbances during menses.

The degree of disturbance depends to a large extent on the individuals outlook towards this physiological and normal process and also on the determination not to allow it to interfere with their normal life. General manifestation such as feeling of lethargy, tiredness, depression, excitability, irritability and even headache, may occur. There is a fullness of breasts. Frequency of urination, constipation or diarrhoea, nausea and vomiting may occur. Some women develop skin rashes and shadows under the eyes.

For pain during menstruation antispasmodic pill such as spasmodon for a day may be taken.

Abnormalities of Menstruation

Menstruation can be inhibited for many months by a subconscious need to attract attention for pregnancy, change in occupation and living conditions. It may be precipitated by excitement. It can become excessive by response to nervous tension and even domestic disharmony.

Amenorrhoea means without or no menses. It may be false or true. It may be false as the girl may be menstruating but due to congenital abnormality blood is not flowing out.

Pseudo or false pregnancy: A sterile woman can have no menses and all the signs of pregnancy but examination and investigation show no pregnancy.

Patient imagines she is pregnant and develops amenorrhoea, nausea, vomiting, swelling of the abdomen.

Similarly changes of climate, occupation and living conditions can cause amenorrhoea. Work involving institutional life, long hours of study and worry over examination is prone to have this effect.

Pathological Causes: There may be congenital defects of the genital system such as absence of ovaries and uterus, same is true of infection acute or chronic, particularly Tuberculosis, certain drugs, dietary deficiency, during childhood and hormonal imbalance leading to obesity are some of the causes of amenorrhoea.

My advice is, if menstruation has not started by the age of 16 years a doctor may be consulted who can investigate and find the cause of non-menstruation.

Scanty Menses: Due to disfunctioning of various hormones and also nervous and emotional factors, scanty menses can be caused.

In most cases scanty menses characterize the whole of menstrual life of a woman and is to be regarded as an emotional trait of no significance.

Infrequent Menstruation: This can be defined arbitrarily as one in which the cycle lasts longer than 35 days. It may be again due to constitutional, physiological, condition following menarache or preceding menopause.

Menorrhaia: As opposed to scanty menses, there can be excessive bleeding during menses either in amount or duration.

Causes are ovarian dysfunction, tumours of the ovary or uterus or blood diseases.

Again causes also can be psychological upsets, nervous tension, anxiety states, unsatisfied sex urge, marital upsets, overwork and also infection and diabetes. Best is to consult a doctor.

Ten per cent female infants have bleeding from the vagina 2-3 days after birth. An unborn infant receives high levels of ovarian hormones from the mother through the placenta. After birth this process is stopped and the child has bleeding due to withdrawal of the hormone. No treatment is required.

Pubertal Bleeding: This occurs between menarche and some years and could be extremely alarming and persistent. The causes are mostly seen in spoilt, often only children and overconscious parents.

Menopausal or post-menopausal bleeding: with or without amenorrhoea or menstrual irregularity is very sinister. Menstruation continuing after the age of 55 years should be investigated as it can be the first sign of cancer of the uterus.

Dysmenorrhoea: It means painful menses. Not less than 50 per cent women are said to experience some discomfort during menses. 50 per cent of the girls are incapacitated for several hours, or one or two days each month. The incidence is affected by social status, occupation and age.

During and just before menses most women are less efficient physically and more unstable emotionally. These factors alone lower pain threshold and lead to exaggeration of minor discomfort.

The expectation of pain is fostered by an over anxious parent and also by curtailment of normal activities during menses. A dysmenorrhic mother often has a dysmenorrhic daughter.

Treatment: The last hope of limiting the intensity of dysmenorrhoea lies in teaching young girls of proper outlook on menstruation, sex and health in general. So it is necessary to correct unfavourable environmental factors, malnutrition and physical activity. Hot water bag on the abdomen can be kept to lessen the pain. Mild sedatives or pain killers are very useful. Correction of constipation which precedes the onset of menses by taking laxative is very useful and helps in minimizing the pain.

Dysmenorrhoea disappears after childbirth except in very few cases.

Endometriosis: Endometriosis is a condition affecting women which occurs to the cells from the lining membrane of the uterus that is endometrium become piled over and settle down in fallopian tubes, ovaries, in pertonal cavity and behind the uterus. Sometimes after operation of the uterus these cells may settle in abdominal wound and every month during menses there is dark blood seen oozing out from the wound.

Symptoms: Chronic or acute pain during menses, severe dysmenorrhoea, backache pain during intercourse, difficulty while passing stool and also infertility and cyst formation in the abdomen.

Treatment : Consult a doctor. Ultrasonography will confirm the diagnosis. There are drugs that dissolve these cysts, etc.

If the condition is not cured by drugs then operation clearing of the endomentrium from outside the uterus and drugs may cure this condition.

3

MENOPAUSE

Dr. Vatsala Samant

It is a change of life due to cessation of menstruation. It usually occurs between the age of 45 to 52 years. It can manifest by sudden stoppage of menses without any warning, but it is most often heralded by gradual decrease in the amount and frequency of menstruation during several months or even years before complete stoppage of menses. When a woman does not menstruate for one year then only she is said to be having menopause.

Physical Changes

Waist line is lost, obesity sets in. Obesity is due to hormonal imbalance and also due to eating habits. The psychological upset brings fear to do something particularly in the nights which are sleepless. Women eat more and at odd times and add to their weight. Hirsutism or slight growth of hair on face and hands causes embarrassment. Breasts become pendulous or may even shrink. Blood pressure is erratic. There can be frequency of urination, arthritis gastrointestinal disturbances, constipation, diarrhoea, osteoporosis.

Psychological Changes

These changes depend on the make-up of the individual. It is also influenced by certain facts—whether the woman is single and unmarried, if married whether she is childless or even grand childless, whether surrounded by happy family, or a widow with the responsibility of looking after her family or also employed and happy in her profession.

Very often, emotional upset is due to the fact and the feeling that this means end of reproduction, fear of loss of feminity and loss of husband's affection which is particularly exaggerated by old folk. There is also the fear that she is entering cancer era. All this leads to nervous symptoms like depression, irritability inability to concentrate, headache, giddiness, gastrointestinal disturbances, insomnia or sleepless nights.

Palpitation and hot flushes particularly at night may occur. These flushes are short-lived and may end in sweating and leaving the woman bathed in sweat and completely exhausted. A woman who was loving and understanding gets bouts of anger and finds fault on flimsy ground and the whole family scenario is changed.

Management

Assurance to the woman approaching menopause is to explain to them that this is a change of life and not the end of life. Obesity can be prevented by reasonable restricted diet and exercise. It is a challenge to remain fit in mind and body and they should think that this period has a compensation of its own, particularly after the stress of pregnancy and childbirth, this change should bring tranquility and peace. It has been my experience that working in a satisfying profession such as doctors, lawyers, managing directors and even teachers do not suffer from psychological changes. They are busy from morning to evening, dead-tired, and so have no time to think about themselves. There is no insomnia, diet is restricted due to working hours and so no obesity and they are happy with this change of life. The fear of loosing feminity and sex urge is wrong. A woman can have sex if she so desires.

Mild doses of ovarian hormones may be taken after consulting doctor.

Premature Menopause

No treatment is required.

Delayed Menopause

If menses continues after the age of 57 years it is a clear indication to consult a doctor.

Artificial Menopause

Surgical removal of uterus or ovaries, irradiation of the ovaries are the causes of stoppage of menses.

In conclusion many of the symptoms unnecessarily attributed to menopause are due to ageing and not to menopause, such as high blood pressure and heart disease.

It is nature's confirmation that they can no longer bear children and this can make it a landmark of profound physiological significance. For some women it brings a real sense of liberation while others find it depressing and some start feeling negative only to discover gradually the positive end.

Research is continuing on whether to take HRT (Hormone Replacement Therapy) or not. It is an option open to all. In India, except for the rich and elite women, it has not been used to alleviate menopause symptoms. Women having diabetes, liver disease, gall bladder and endometriosis are not fit for HRT. HRT women need counselling and careful clinical management.

At this stage a woman should have such a diet which keeps her blood sugar steady. Taking enough of calcium, particularly in milk and food, reduces risk of osteoporosis. Vitamin C and E are helpful in reducing hot flushes, nervousness, fatigue, insomnia, dizziness, palpitation, etc. Exercise is helpful to allay some symptoms.

Hormone Replacement Therapy

HRT goes back to 1950 when estrogen an ovarian hormone was prescribed for hot flushes, sweats, vaginal dryness, joint discomfort and urinary problems. In 1960, it became clear that estrogen on its own was not the answer. Just taking estrogen increases the risk of endometrial hyperplasia which causes thickening of the lining of the uterus, a forerunner of uterine cancer. A small quantity of progestogen was added to estrogen.

HRT is being taken by 80 per cent women in America and Canada for menopausal symptoms. It can be taken as a pill, applied as skin cream, skin patches implants, a vaginal cream or pesbary. Some doctors favour HRT as soon as women are over 70 to avoid osteoporosis or thinning of the bones.

Drawbacks

If only estrogen is taken it increases the risk of breast cancer. Progestogen with estrogen promotes the return of periods and can bring back pre-menopausal syndrome with bleeding bouts mood changes and breast tenderness.

4

BREAST

Dr. Vatsala Samant

Development, Function and Disorders

At birth breasts are small and in female infant nipples are slightly larger than in the males. Breasts begin to enlarge by the age of nine years and within the next two to three years fat is deposited and breasts become round and prominent.

During menstrual cycle breasts also undergo a cyclical change. They may increase in size a weak before menses and some women complain of pain. After menses, pain and enlargement disappear.

During pregnancy breasts enlarge, nipples become pigmented and there is a watery discharge from the nipples. After delivery there is activity in the breast and on the third day of delivery a thick yellowish substance known as colostrum is secreted from the nipples. Milk is secreted from the fourth day onwards and sucking by the child helps in more secretion of milk.

Breasts are meant to provide best nutrition to the child and are under the control of ovarian and other hormones.

Abnormalities

Various, degrees of underdevelopment of the breasts are seen, particularly in those who have to work on stage and as models. They seek medical advice for the same.

Causes and Remedies

Deficiency of ovarian hormones and diet are the causes. The patient should increase her weight, have physiotherapy and local massage. Exercise of pectoral muscles and small doses of hormones prescribed by the doctors may help these patients. Plastic surgery is done and fat is deposited in the breast.

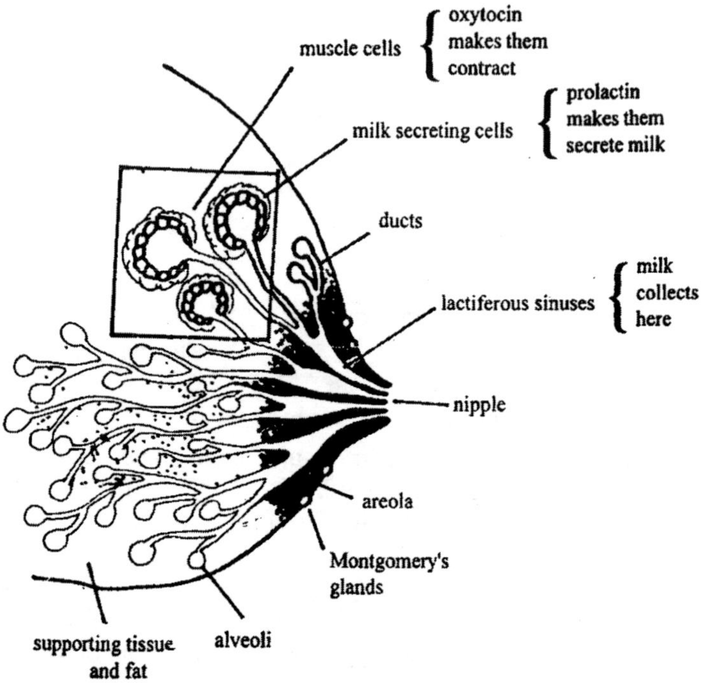

Fig. 1: Anatomy of the Breast.

Asymmetrical Breasts

Even though the two breasts appear similar, no two breasts are similar unless the dissimilarity is very obvious nothing should be done.

Accessory Breasts and Nipples

In many women there is a prolongation of the breast gland to the axilla known as axillary tail. This may enlarge during menstrual cycle, and lactation, and cause pain and lump.

Sometimes there are extra axillary nipples along the abdomen as in animals and they are harmless.

Pendulous Breasts

Cause is unknown and are first noticed at puberty. There are reports of increase by 6-13 kg. Breasts become pendulous after lactation, advancing age and general obesity, treatment is good support.

Gynaecomastitis

female babies. There may be even discharge from the nipples popularly known as witches milk. It is due to the stoppage of hormone from the mother after birth. No treatment is required and the swelling disappears during the course of time.

Mastitis

It is common after delivery and during purperium sometime resulting in abscess formation requiring incision, and is due to cracked nipples.

Chronic Mastitis

Women in their forties and fifties complain of mammary discomfort. Breasts become tender and have an undefined nodularity. Women are afraid that this nodular swelling may be precursor of cancer. Ultrasound mammography is done these days to rule out malignancy.

Acute Mastitis

There is another type of mastitis or inflamation of the breast particularly after delivery during purperium. This is due to cracked nipples. Breasts get infected and may form breast abscess. Breasts become painful and tender, there is swelling with redness, fever and general malaise. Treatment is surgical. Incision of the abscess and stoppage of lactation from the infected breasts.

Tumours

Non-malignant tumours such as fibroadenoma of the breasts are quite common, even amongst young girls and must be surgically removed and sent for histopathology. Malignant tumours, or cancer of the breasts is discussed in the chapter on Cancer.

Galactorrhea

Prolactin a secretion of pituitary gland stimulates the breast glands to produce milk and enables the mother to nurse her child. Physiological increase of prolactin occurs only in pregnancy, Galactorrhea is a term to describe pathological discharge of milk from the breasts at any time other than pregnancy. Patients suffering from galactorrhea are infertile and there may be stoppage of menses. It can be present in men also. This condition is due to increase of prolactin which may be due to a tumour of pituitary gland. Investigation either by X-ray of the skull or CAT scan and estimation of prolactin should be done. This condition can be completely cured by medication. I had a patient with galactorrhea and infertility. After proper treatment ovulation producing drug was given which resulted in pregnancy. She gave birth to twins. After a year or so she suffered from galactorrhea but now it is under control.

5

CONCEPTION

Dr. Vatsala Samant

The science of pregnancy, childbirth and care of the mother is called obstetrics. In short, liberated ripe egg, mated by a spermatozoa and fertilized is the precursor of a child. Semen (man's reproductive discharge) is deposited in the vagina of the female. There are thousands of sperms ejaculated in the vagina. Most of them die. Only few enter the uterus through the cervix. They travel through the fallopian tube and reach uterus. Only one sperm is allowed to enter it by penetration and looses its head and tail and the nuclei of the sperm and ovum form a single nucleous forerunner of the child to be. This fertilized ovum travels back through the tube to the uterus to be embedded. The hormones of ovary and uterus are prepared to receive the ovum, protect it and nourish it till the placenta is formed. The size of the uterus increases from 2 grams to 2 pounds.

There is new muscle formation and dilation of the blood vessels and better blood supply. Pregnancy is a natural and physiological event but it is also a period of stress and strain for the woman. It can temporarily alter the whole outlook of a woman. In early months depression, irritability, emotional instability, lethargy are all common symptoms.

During the mid term months there is a feeling of well-being and the woman is full of energy. She is placid and happy. Just before labour, she is definitely uncomfortable. Labour or childbirth is a period of exhaustion and agony. After birth of the child, exhaustion turns into exhilaration and agony in to ecstacy. Mother feels relieved and happy on hearing the cry of baby.

Signs and Symptom

Fifty per cent of the women suffer from nausea and vomiting because of amenorrhoea or no menses. There are changes in the breasts, enlargement, discolouration of nipples and watery discharge, abdomen starts getting bigger. Fat is deposited in various parts of the body.

Extra Uterine Pregnancy

Sometimes pregnancy ends abruptly. Natural habitat of an embryo is the uterus but sometimes due to obstruction in the tube the egg does not reach the uterus and starts growing in the fallopian tubes or even ovary. Tube is thin walled and incapable of nourishing the ovum with the result that the tube rupture and the ovum dies and forms a lump and tube tries to throw it in the abdomen. This causes internal bleeding, excruciating pain and shock. Very rarely foetus survives after rupture. It gets attached to the intestines and develops, but ultimately dies inside the abdomen. The only remedy in Extra Uterine Pregnancy is surgery of the abdomen and removing the foetus. Signs and symptoms vary according to the condition. There may or may not be history of Amenorrhoea and during the catastrophe there may be bleeding or no bleeding from the vagina. There may be excessive pain, abdominal distension and signs of internal bleeding. It is a very serious problem and immediate surgery and blood transfusion only can save the patient.

I remember a case when I was a medical superintendent. A woman was admitted with excruciating pain, tender abdominal enlargement. Her mother pointed out to me that she had borne five children but during this pregnancy she used to complain of attacks of pain during her nine months and fainting attacks too. Those were the days of no blood transfusion, no sonography and anaesthesia and my nurses used to give ether anesthesia. Clinical diagnosis confirmed extra uterine full term pregnancy and on opening the abdomen the diagnosis was confirmed, child was dead and the patient died of internal haemorrage.

I have myself suffered from Ectopic pregnancy. I had to fly to Bombay where I was operated at the K.E.M. Hospital. My condition was so bad that the anaesthetic told the surgeon to hurry up to avoid DOT (Death On Table) but I survived. On another occasion in Allahabad on the hottest day of June I had to go to see a patient who had suddenly collapsed. As her husband was not available I brought her to the clinic and confirmed my diagnosis of Ectopic Pregnancy and operated on her without the presence of her husband. We had to give her two bottles of blood. She survived and is perfectly alright.

6

DEVELOPMENT OF THE EMBRYO

Dr. Vatsala Samant

The most rapid growth in a human being's life is when a single microscopic cell develops into a full grown baby. This takes place during pregnancy. Changes in a growing baby are reflected in its mother. The hormones act as chemical messages from the unborn child to its mother. These messages are passed in the mother's body where they affect her—mentally, emotionally and physically.

The embryo is formed by a fusion of a sperm (from the father) and an ovum (from the mother). In 38 weeks, that single cell multiplies to more than 6 million cells. The embryo begins to develop in the uterus and by eight weeks most of its organs are already appearing and the embryo begins to resemble a human being. By 14 weeks all the limbs and internal organs are formed and development is then by growth only. At this stage the embryo (foetus) is a miniature human being.

For the first 28 days, there is little sexual difference in the outside of the embryo. By the fifth week the effects of the sex chromozomes on the embryonic baby start to show. Either a penis and a prostate gland develop, or a pair of fallopian tubes and a uterus.

The baby makes himself known by 22-24 weeks, the baby in the womb has grown to the extent that his mother is aware of his presence. He moves frequently, stretching his limbs, back and head so that 'kicking' is not felt just where the legs are, but all over the stomach. There is still a lot of fluid around the developing baby so that he can move around. Most babies by this stage of pregnancy settle in a head down position but 10-20 per cent will still be wandering. There is no harm in this, and most of the wanderers will be in the head down position by 34-36 weeks. Twenty-eight weeks is the legally accepted time at which the baby is considered capable of surviving outside the womb. Many babies who are born at this stage grow to be physically and mentally normal; but, ideally, it is better for the unborn child to mature in the womb for another ten weeks.

Care for Mother after Childbirth

It is very important for the mother to become fit after childbirth. Then only she can take proper care of the child and resume her everyday activities. For that she must do exercise as the pelvic floor muscles and abdominal muscles become very stretched.

The pelvic floor muscles surround the anus, vagina and urethra tube through which urine is passed from the bladder. They support the contents of the pelvis, the womb, the bladder and the bowel.

If these become weak then there can be serious problems.

The abdominal muscles support the abdominal organs and the spine. After childbirth the stretched and weakened muscles often cause backache.

To tone up and strengthen the affected muscles the following exercises should be performed.

Exercise for Pelvic Floor Muscles

Clench and draw in the muscles in and around your anus and vagina. Continue to clench the muscles while counting slowly up to four. Relax, pause and repeat four times. At first you may not be able to get beyond a count of one. But by the third or fourth day after childbirth you should be able to do the full count without causing strain. The exercise is performed at hourly intervals during the day in the following three positions:

Exercise for the Abdominal Muscles

Exercise One

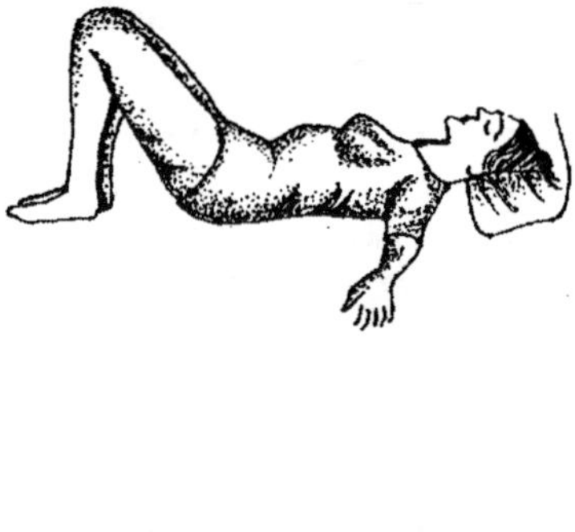

Lie on your back with your knees bent, your feet flat and your arms outstretched at your sides. Clench your buttocks and simultaneously draw in your abdominal muscles. Continue until the small of your back is pressed against the floor or bed and then relax. Perform the exercise five times running, twice a day, building upto 20 times running, twice a day.

Exercise Two

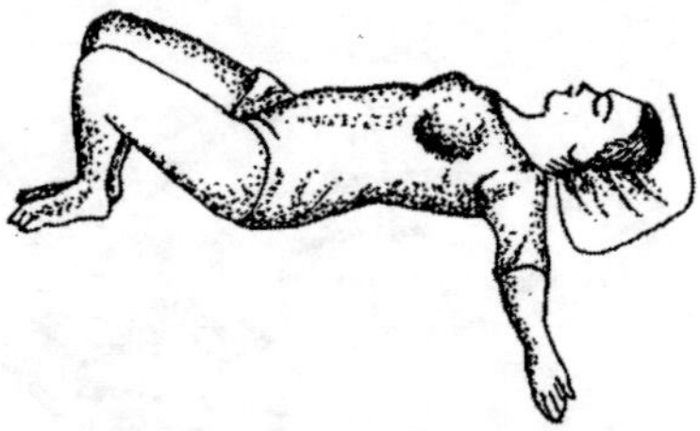

Lie on your back with your knees bent, your feet flat and your arms outstretched at your sides. Tilt your pelvis backwards. Put your heels and ankles close together. Then swing your knees as far as possible to one side.

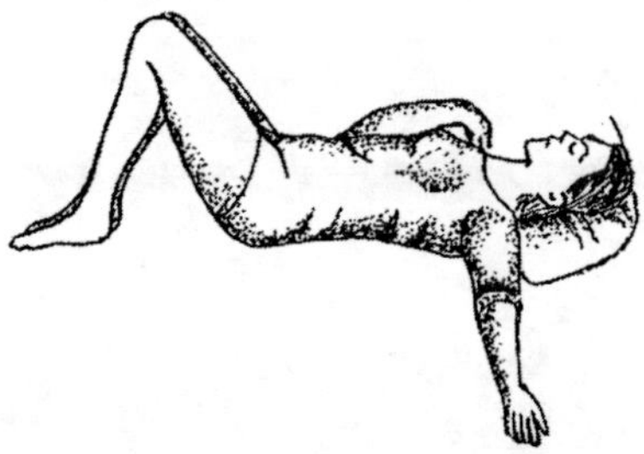

Return to your original position, relax and repeat to the other side. Perform the exercise five times running, twice a day, building up to 20 times running.

Exercice Three

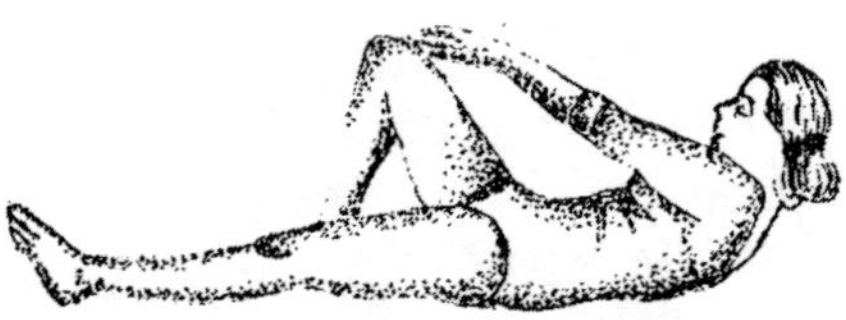

Lie on your back with your right leg straight, your left leg bent and your arms outstretched at your sides. Tilt your pelvis backwards. Then lift your head and touch your left knee with your right hand.

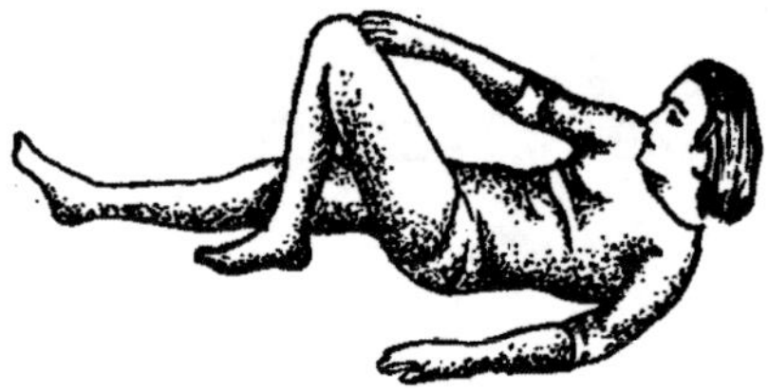

Relax and repeat to the other side. Perform the exercise five times running, twice a day, building up to 20 times running.

7

PREGNANCY

Dr. Vatsala Samant

Every woman desires motherhood— a most vital function she has to perform. It is a natural function but it certainly is a period of stress and strain. It is the mother who nourishes the baby, protects the unborn from heat and cold for a period of nine months. After childbirth she has to feed the baby, look after his or her welfare. All this causes strain on the mother and even though she is performing a natural function, she may have to pay the price of becoming disabled or even face death.

Maternal death is very high in India. In developed countries it has been reduced to minimum.

Antenatal care is absolutely necessary to rule out chronic diseases like tuberculosis, heart diseases, etc., before deciding to enter motherhood. Premarital examination is one of the methods of finding out these diseases.

Antenatal Care

Once pregnancy has taken place, it is necessary to have a check up particularly to rule out anaemia, high blood pressure and diabetes. In the beginning a check up should be done every month and mid trimester every fifteen days and later on every week. Undue increase in the weight is one of the signs of Toximiao also presence of Albumin in the urine. Blood Pressure check up is very important. During antenatal care, the doctors try to find out how the baby is growing and its position in the uterus. The mother should take correct and nutritious diet. A mother is not supposed to eat double the quantity, but simple nourishing diet like milk, milk products, fruits, pulses, etc., at short intervals.

To facilitate natural birth certain relaxing exercises are taught. During antenatal care, previously existing diseases like those of heart are detected and treated.

Object of antenatal care is to reduce toll of maternity and give a healthy child to a healthy mother. Antenatal care has been the best weapon to reduce maternal mortality. It has achieved wonders in the Western countries. In India there are two types of patients—educated women who take the benefit of ANC and uneducated who neglect themselves till the labour pain starts, and pay the price or toll of maternity. A woman must consult a doctor as early as possible when she is pregnant.

Often Tetanus infects the mother and newborn infant and so treatment against Tetanus is a must.

Anaemia and High Blood Pressure are detected and the greater weight of the expecting mother is a parameter to detect the growth of the unborn and also undue weight gain of the mother to be.

Infections particularly HIV and German Measles which lead to deform the unborn baby can be detected at an early stage. Ultrasonography is good to detect abnormalities of the foetus.

Childbirth

Childbirth depends on three factors—passage of the mother through which an infant is to be born, passenger or the unborn baby, and last but very important is uterine action or force with which it can expel the infant. First two factors, passage and passenger can be predicted in the antenatal clinic, but the last can only be assessed once the pain start. Normal delivery is the aim of all practicing doctors, if all the three factors are normal. There can be no natural delivery without pain. There are pain killers but they may harm the baby to be born and sometimes even the mother.

A baby can be born naturally or by operative procedure known as caesarean and forceps delivery.

During normal delivery there is bound to be some sort of injury to the perinium and to avoid bad tears, a clean cut is given on the perinium and stitched with care.

During the post-natal period, uterus which weighed 2 ounces has to grow to 2 pounds to accommodate the infant and forces it out with muscular contractions. After delivery, the uterus reduces and goes back to its normal size. This process takes 40 days.

After delivery breasts are set in action—milk is produced by ovarian hormone. Bleeding from the uterus may continue for a month or so but if it is profuse then the doctor may be consulted. It may be due to infection or retained some product or placenta retained in uterus after delivery.

Post-Natal Care or Puerperium

Post-natal care is necessary to see that the mother is taking sufficient nourishment and rest. During pregnancy a woman puts on weight and during puerperium she has to reduce it by some kind of simple exercises. She cannot afford to go on a lean diet as she has to nurse the baby.

Placenta site in the uterus is a raw area and prone to infection. Great hygienic care has to be taken to avoid sepsis. The *Dai* does not observe aseptic methods in conducting a delivery and mother may die if puerperal sepsis sets in. Fever, pus discharge from the vagina are some of the symptoms. Antibiotics have reduced the incidence of sepsis.

RH Factor

We have our blood in four groups— A, B, AB and O. Besides these, there is a factor RH or Rhesus factor, an antigen which was discovered in 1940 is present in the red cells. People whose RBC contains this RH antigen are said to be RH Positive and people in whom this factor is not present are known to be RH Negative. An infant inherits either father's or mother's blood group. If the mother is RH Negative and father RH Positive there is every chance of the child being RH Positive. If the mother is RH Negative and unborn child RH Positive Antibodies are formed in mother's blood and these antibodies enter the foetus through placenta and destroy the red blood cells of the foetus causing anaemia, jaundice and even death of foetus in the uterus. During the first pregnancy the foetus is not affected but in the second pregnancy foetus is definitely affected if RH Positive.

During antenatal care if mother is RH Negative antibody titre of mother's blood is assessed and treatment is given. The infant of a RH Negative is assessed for Red Blood Cell count, jaundice and treated by the pediatrician and mother is given routine injection Rholin within 48 hours of delivery to prevent second baby from suffering jaundice, etc. RH Negative mother does not suffer from RH Negative Blood but it is the baby who suffers if RH Positive. RH Negative person—man or woman cannot receive RH Positive blood transfusion except in an emergency.

8

PROBLEMS DURING PREGNANCY

Dr. Vatsala Samant

Sex of the Baby

At conception only the sex of the baby is determined. Ovum carries X chromosomes and the sperm carries both X and Y chromosomes. The ovum and sperm chromosomes are joined. If both chromosomes are XX a female child is conceived but if they are XY a male child is conceived.

Problems during Pregnancy

The first symptoms of pregnancy are nausea and vomiting.

The pregnant woman should take small snacks like biscuits, etc. Nausea and vomiting finishes by the twelfth or fourteenth week of pregnancy.

Breathlessness

As the mother's weight increases, her heart has to work harder. Oxygen is also required by the growing baby in the womb and so it makes more demands on her heart. A healthy woman may not be affected although she may notice palpitations and breathlessness at slight exertion. This is normal as the growing uterus is pressing up on the underside of the lungs and there is less space to breathe.

Heartburn

The expanding uterus forces some of the acid contents into the gullet where it produces heart burn. It can be treated with mild antacids.

Piles

There is a pressure inside the abdomen, and because of that varicose veins (piles) form around the anus. Constipation makes the condition worse to avoid it one should drink plenty of water and eat dietary fibre, beans, salads and green vegetables or take a mild laxative.

Varicose veins first form spidery groups of thin blue lines on the thighs. They disappear after the baby is born. The larger varicose veins are soft knot like swellings formed by the enlargement of the veins. They can occur inside the thighs and vulva.

During the third trimester of pregnancy fluid retention can lead to ocdemia visible in the ankles, feet, hands and face of the pregnant woman.

Fatigue

The tiredness so often experienced in the first trimester is usually less noticeable in the middle trimester but becomes increasingly severe towards. the last days. It is necessary to have some rest after having lunch.

Insomnia

Many women experience problems of sleeplessness as their pregnancy progresses. They are uncomfortable and cannot find satisfactory sleeping positions. Some fall asleep but are unable to sleep again after many times going to the toilet. The psychological changes of pregnancy and impending labour pain and motherhood gives rise to anxieties, fears and worries in the pregnant woman. Relaxation has a very important solution of insomnia when the woman is unable to get sleep, she should eat something after that she can have a warm drink and then go back to bed and try to sleep in a comfortable and well supported position. This can solve the insomnia problem without resorting to sleeping pills.

Back and pelvis pain may occur at any time but is more common between the fourth and seventh months.

9

ABORTION

Dr. Vatsala Samant

Termination of pregnancy is known as abortion. Incidence of abortion is about 20 per cent. There are many causes of abortion.

Symptoms

There is bleeding from the vagina. Initially it is scanty but later on it starts bleeding profusely. There is pain during childbirth, quite excruciating painful abdominal spasms.

Treatment depends on the type of abortion and best thing is to leave it to the doctor.

What is missed abortion? There is a history of Ammenorhoea. Slight bleeding and pain may be there which subsides in a day or two. The embryo of the child dies but it remains in the uterus. Sonography confirms the diagnosis and is very useful. Treatment is to evacuate the uterus by D&C or dilation of the cervix and cleaning the uterus.

Habitual Abortion

Two or three successive abortions mostly due to genetic causes are known as habitual abortion. As a rule habitual abortion is spontaneous.

Criminal Abortion

An induced abortion and that also criminally not therapeutically or legally, is known as Criminal Abortion.

Abortion is practiced by all kinds of medical and non-medical persons and has not done away with criminal abortion. Criminal abortion is dangerous because it is practiced by quacks or semi-skilled individuals and that also under unhygienic conditions. These are performed in secrecy. Domestic instruments, hairpins, bark of a tree, knitting needles, chemicals and dirty cloth pieces are inserted in vagina. The result is infection and injury to the vagina and uterus. Many women die of septic abortion or become disabled and sterile.

Liberalization of abortion law and medical termination of pregnancy has been passed by the parliament, even to the extent of allowing termination on demand and is practiced all over India.

Therapeutic Abortion

Abortion is induced where there is a pressing indication in the interest of the mother. There are many indications like heart and lung disease, kidney syndrome, etc. The doctor has to decide whether induction of abortion or continuation of pregnancy is beneficial to the mother or not. Rubella or German Measles affect the unborn child causing various congenital deformities. It can be distinguished by blood test. Generally, according to famous obstetricians pregnancy should be terminated in such cases.

10

CHILD BIRTH—LABOUR

Dr. Vatsala Samant

Normally a baby is born after forty weeks of gestation. Sometimes the baby may be born before 36 weeks of gestation and is naturally a premature baby.

Childbirth is achieved by a process known as labour; and labour is achieved by contractions of uterine and abdominal muscles and is divided into three stages.

First Stage

Labour may start with show, i.e., discharge of blood and mucus from the vagina or sometimes by early rupture of the *liquar amnia* (dry labour). The uterine contractions to begin with are every 20 minutes or so, lasting for a few seconds. Gradually they increase in rythym and last longer and are very painful. The purpose of contraction is to dilate the cervical opening and reduce the upper part of the womb so that the foetus is pushed down into the vagina. This goes on till the cervix is fully dilated. If the bag of water is present it can be seen at the vulval opening, quite often the bag bursts or is punctured by the doctor and the first stage is completed.

Second Stage

The contractions of the abdominal muscles begins. Uterine contractions are strong and more painful and there is an urge to defecate. Anus also is dilated. In a normal delivery the baby is delivered—the head comes out first and the body follows. To avoid bad tears of the vagina and perenium an incision known as episiotomy is done under local anesthesia.

Third Stage

Uterus takes a little rest and allows placenta to separate from the uterine mucosa and is ready for expulsion, a few uterine contractions and slight pull on the umbilical cord and little bleeding, placenta is expelled. An injection to contract the uterus is given so that there should be no extra bleeding and the episiotomy wound is stitched.

Cause of labour is not known. Duration of labour varies from person to person and is longer in primipara (first baby) than in multipara.

Pain in Labour

There can be no normal delivery without pain. Every pregnant woman has to go though the ordeal of labour pains. During the first stage, relaxation techniques and mild analgesics may relieve the pain to a certain extent. In the second stage, mild whips of anesthesia and caudal injection may be used but these methods may harm the baby. Pain is a symptom which differs from person to person—their outlook, personality and previous experience of labour. For a mother the first sight of the baby blots out all memories of labour pain. Unfortunately there will be some women who will always grumble and say they can never forget the ordeal of labour pains even after many many years.

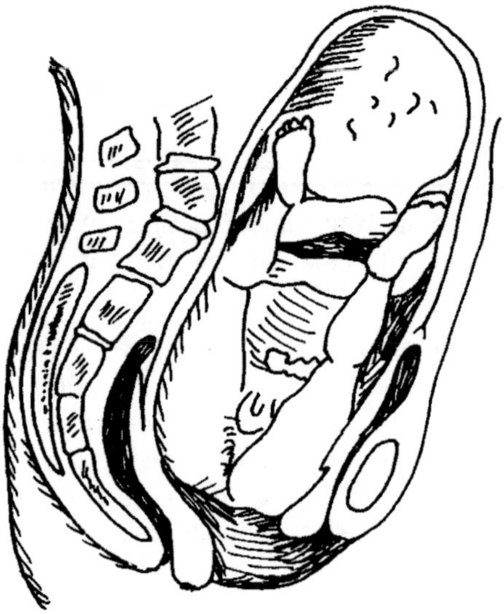

Breech

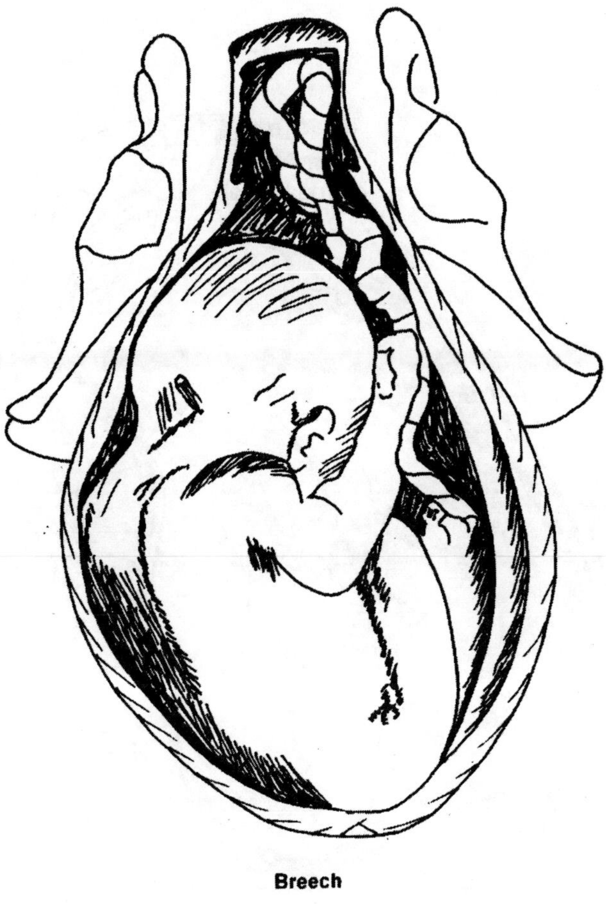

Breech

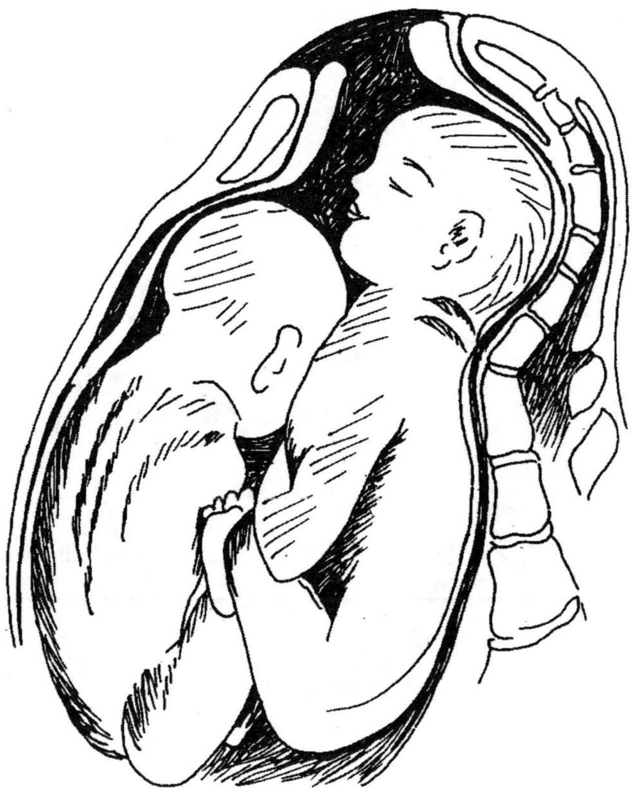

Twins

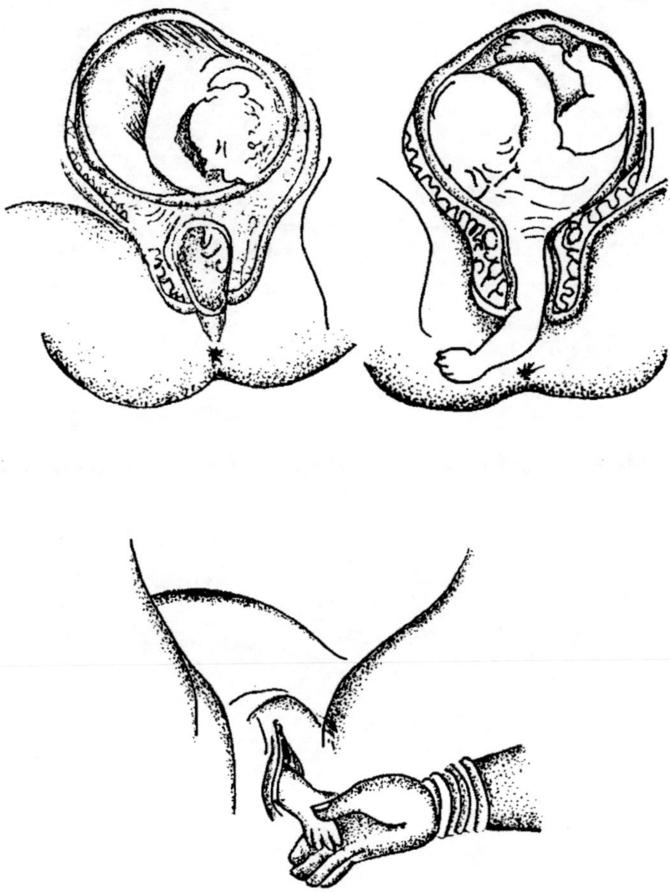

Transverse lie and Hand Prolapse

11

RCH–REPRODUCTIVE CHILD HEALTH

Dr. Vatsala Samant

India has 16 per cent or 1/6th of the world population and is going to have one billion people of its own soon to come. In 1951, India was the first country in the world to start working (officially) a programme on family planning. Hospitals, government and other were to start family planning clinics, with Intrauterine devices, Tubectomy or sterilization, etc. Kamla Nehru Hospital received reward for doing excellent work in this programme. Soon the programme remained a voluntary programme.

To lenovate the programme Familly Planning become family welfare but most of the programme remains on paper.

Now a new approach to the all important issue and population stabilization is under way for quite some time since 1977. Family welfare or family planning has been names as RCH reproductive Child health Programme. RCH aims that health of the mother and child is looked after efficiently and it upto for small family norm "Hum Do Hamare Do". To make reproduction a healthy affair there should be an awareness about sexually transmited diseases like syphilis, gonorrhoea and AIDS. S.T.D. affects 90 per cent of the population. I know a case of a young 18-year old boy working as a servant was suffering from gonorrhoea and he had indulged in sex with prostitute.

To make the programme successful women must be freed from all forms of coercion, discrimination, violence and should be educated and must be free and responsible decision about their sexuality reproductive health and decide when to have a baby and safe pregnancy. About 9000 mothers die during pregnancy and childbirth. Couples must be taught to have sexual relationship without facing and fear of pregnancy, in short to have a baby by choice and not by chance when couples health, economic conditions can bring up the child with love and makes a good citizen of India.

Population growth is now reduced turn 2 per cent per annum to 1.8 in number a drop in the occure. Maternal and infant mortality rate is also reduced even than immunization, RCH, etc., there is no apprecable check on population growth in India. Our population a large segment of youth who are ignorant of healthy sexual life and unfortunately there is no political and religious commitment regarding RCH. While countries like Malasiya and Thailand have been successful on checking population explosion.

12

HAZARDS OF PUERPERIUM AND POST-NATAL PERIOD

Dr. Vatsala Samant

Puerperium is the period between childbirth and return of the womb to its normal state, usually about 6 weeks.

Post-natal is period immediately after childbirth.

There are many problems which arise during these periods.

Pelvic and abdominal muscles surround the anus, vagina and urethra and also the contents of the pelvis uterus bladder and bowels and when weakened they can cause urinary trouble and uterine prolapse.

During puerperium the woman can suffer disabilities, retention of urine or incontinuance of urine because the perinium (private part) is sore. There is an episiotomy wound which causes these discomforts. Treatment for retention of urine is catheterization of the bladder for 1 or 2 days and then educating her to pass urine by herself. Constipation and piles is a very common complaint during puerperium. It is due to the painful episiotomy and the fear of the wound opening out, that the mother is afraid of passing stool and thus suffers constipation.

It is also due to weakness of the abdominal muscles and change in diet which is enforced after delivery. Constipation gives rise to piles and bleeding.

Episiotomy wound can become painful and swollen and even infected. Infrared radiation, warm saline baths or ice packs may relieve the pain.

During ten days of puerperium there can be secondary haemorrhage from the uterus. This is due to retained placental bits and membrane or infection of the uterus. This is a very serious condition and requires immediate hospitalization and even blood transfusion.

Haematoma or collection of blood in the vagina or perinium which gives rise to severe pain at the back. Internal examination should be done. Treatment is incision and packing.

Backpain which is a constant complaint throughout pregnancy and then during post-natal period may be severe due to injury to the bone cocyx or lumber vertebrae and their joints. Some women suffer from after pains due to contractions of the uterus particularly while lactacting.

Fatigue can be harrassing in the early days after childbirth due to baby feeding every three hours and not getting enough rest and sleep. Mother should adjust her daily lifestyle in such a way that she should get enough rest and sleep, and here the husband can be of great help by looking after the baby when the mother is resting.

Breasts due to cracked nipples can develop breast abscess which may require incision.

Psycosis is a condition known as puerperal insanity. Women become agitated, anxious, depressed, exhausted and may not be able to sleep or eat which can lead to weakness. Sometimes she can become violent requiring hospitalization.

Puerperal sepsis infection of the genital track due to unhygienic conditions is also a serious problem. There is high fever and pain. Foul vaginal discharge comes out and if not treated in time the patient can die. These days this problem can be treated with the help of antibiotics.

13

TOLL OF MATERNITY

Dr. Vatsala Samant

Women have to perform the most vital function of motherhood. Many women die during childbirth. Certain type of hens die after producing eggs similarly eels die after giving birth to little ones in Bermuda. This is known as maternal mortality. In India maternal mortality is very high, while in developed countries, particularly in the West it has been reduced to a minimum.

It took a long time to start antenatal clinics in India. In big cities like Delhi, Mumbai, Chennai and Calcutta clinics were opened. Women from rural areas were brought to the hospital in dying conditions handled by local *dai* and it usually ended in death of the patient. Even now, regular scientific antenatal care is lacking particularly amongst the rural population. Antenatal care should start early in pregnancy to detect existing diseases, such as, heart disease, tuberculosis and anaemia which is endemic in our country. Women should be informed about personal hygiene, proper nutrition, etc. The check-up should be every month. Pregnancy is a period of stress and strain, particularly for the kidney, patients and can result in High Blood Pressure. High Blood Pressure can kill the unborn infant and also the mother, so checking the blood pressure is must during pregnancy. Tetanus used to take a high toll. The infant has a wound in the umbilical cord cut and mother a raw area in the uterus placental sight, because of this, the chances of Tetanus become more.

To prevent this disease, tetanus vaccine is given during the antenatal period. Certain amount of weight is gained during pregnancy almost to the tune of 20 lbs. There can be abnormal weight gain due to kidney disfunction and weight checking during the antenatal check this can be detected and treated.

Antenatal check-ups find out whether the baby is growing, its position in the womb and amount of fluid for the foetus to move about ultrasonography has helped in deciding all the facts and has helped in deciding the type of delivery normal or operative even before the woman goes into labour.

Proper antenatal care during pregnancy is must. If the mother is suffering from anaemia or infections or any other disease then it can be detected and treated in time. Nutritious diet and mild exercises are advised. High risk pregnancy treated has reduced the toll of maternity. The aim of antenatal care is to give a healthy child to a healthy mother.

14

FAMILY PLANNING

Dr. Vatsala Samant

Family planning or planned parenthood means having children when parents want them. It does not mean birth control. Birth control is one aspect of family planning. It has wider and higher meaning than just birth control. It has a quantitative and qualitative aspect. The first means regulating the size of family and the proper spacing (gap) of the children. It means that the parents have children when they want them and can afford to have them which connotes when the health of the parents can afford them. Though health depends to large extent on wealth. Family planning also means helping the childless to have children, for a family without children is like a kingdom without people. Spacing of the children or having them at proper interval is also an important aspect of family planning. A child needs a playmate more or less of its own age and too long an interval between one child and the other may be psychologically bad for a child, while too short an interval is very harmful for the growth of the child which is bound to be neglected by the parents. We can just imagine the plight of the parents who have a baby added every year and the model is bound to be defective. This is the qualitative aspect of Family Planning. It means teaching parents how to have healthier children who can become good citizens and be a credit to their family.

In India every year there are 1,50,000 mothers dying in child birth. 20 mothers in every 1,000 die due to child bearing. About 13,000 babies out of one million that are born every year die during the first year of their existence. The sum total maternal and infant deaths during the first year of birth amounts to about three million deaths every year. The picture is not complete, about three millions mothers suffer from permanent or temporary disability resulting from pregnancy or labour. In India, infant mortality is highest because maternal health is poor and consequently children are undernourished and prematurely born. They come in such quick succession that the mother has not had the time to recoup her health from the previous pregnancy. There are many causes of this heavy maternal mortality. Besides, malnutrition, poverty and ignorance, there is one single cause which is responsible for this loss of mothers in multiparity or having too many children at too short interval. It has been proved that maternal mortality sharply rises after the mother gives birth to many children.

It is clear from the above that family planning is a very important means of reducing maternal and infant mortality and preserving health of mothers and children. To obtain the optimum conditions for childbirth it is necessary that mother or both parents must know-how to space their children or have knowledge of family planning and contraception. Birth control is only a new aspect of an age old attempt on the part of the people to solve for themselves the family size. Modern research has made it possible to control conception through the agency of contraceptions.

For such people after they have had all their children lasting or permanent protection against pregnancy can be given by operation or sterlization. These operations can be done an either a man or woman. In woman a part of fallopian tube on either side is removed. No organ is removed. There is no lessening of sex desire and it can be done without risk, within 3 to 4 days of delivery. In men vasectomy or tying the duct is even a simpler procedure than the operation in women. These two methods are best suited for our masses. We should feel proud that Indian Government has adopted planned parenthood as a National and Official Policy. Clinics have been established all over the country.

Family planning improves maternal and infant health and promotes family welfare. It removes the economic distress. It is neither sinful nor immoral. People should take full advantage of these scientific methods, have few but healthier children.

15

CONTRACEPTION

Dr. Manju Varma, M.S.

Population is always in a dynamic state. World's population is increasing by 100 million every year. India with its 25 per cent of world's land accommodates 15 per cent of total population. The industrialized developed world with a sound income per person, has a population doubling time of more than 130 years, while in India if population will keep growing at the present rate it will double in just 35 years. Every year 1.5 million is added to the existing population. This has a direct impact on growing needs and statistically will require:

(i) 10 million tonnes of grains

(ii) 190 million metres of cloth

iii) 03 million dwelling units

(iv) 127,000 schools

(v) 373,000 teachers

(vi) 12,000 beds in hospital

(vii) 4 million jobs.

In addition "too many and too frequent" pregnancies predispose to an increased risk of death of one mother and one new born with more chances of ill-health of both. Parents are unable to provide proper care, love, attention and education to their children. There are increased chances of certain type of cancers, e.g., cervix and also chances of malnourished babies.

The advantages of "Planned Small Family" are very many like, the mother has sufficient time to replenish her depleted body nutrients. There is more time and energy to give proper attention and love to children. Child is also benefited by getting proper nutrition, education and parental love and care. The father is also less burdened and relaxed to provide better food, education, shelter and comforts, etc.

Small families also result in upliftment of community and in improving the living standards. There is a conservation of natural resources. Other burdens are less and there will be less unemployment. Planned Small Families would gradually bring, happiness, peace, harmony and prosperity to individuals and to the nation.

In present century, in addition to other goals we will enter with a concept of "Family Health". The health of the family revolves round the women of the house. From this evolved the current concept of "Reproductive Health" meaning thereby. A State of complete physical, mental and social well-being from puberty to menopause and not merely absence of disease or infirmity in all matters" (WHO, 1994). It includes in addition to Contraception, safe motherhood and child survival, management of infertility (no issues), sexual health and prevention and therapy of carcinom of breast and other reproductive organs.

Woman is the fulcrum of population issues. If we want to ward off the ill-effects of population explosion we have to accept:

(i) Delaying the 1st child

(ii) Keeping an interval of 3-4 years, between two pregnancies

(iii) Having only two children and accepting "Small Family" norms.

This can only be achieved by practice of:

(i) Spacing or temporary methods of family limitation, or

(ii) Limitation of family by permanent methods.

Spacing Methods

Temporary

(i) Intra uterine contraceptive devices

(ii) Steroidal contraceptives

(iii) Non-steroidal contraceptives

(iv) Barrier and chemical contraceptives

(v) Natural methods.

Permanent

(i) Male— Vasectomy

(ii) Female— Tubectomy.

Spacing Methods

Intra Uterine Contraceptive Devices

These devices are Cu-T (Govt.), Multiload, etc. Nova-T are made of special plastic with copper wound around it. This prevents the egg and the sperms from joining and not allowing nidation in uterus. This is inserted by a trained health worker. It cannot be used by women with history of abnormal or irregular or heavy bleeding during menses, H/o tube pregnancy. The provider also has to exclude infection of reproductive organs, abnormalities, tumour or injury of uterus.

It should ideally be inserted just after the menses. It can also be given after abortion. The lady should be trained to feel the thread. She should come back for follow up after 1 month and then after 3 months thereafter every 6 and 12 months for 3-4 years when it has to be changed. This temporary method should be used for spacing of children.

Steroidal Contraceptives

Pill: It contains oestrogen and progesterone hormone in low dosage. These hormones stop women's ovary from releasing egg, so she cannot become pregnant. It is supplied by the government free of cost under Family Welfare Programme as 21 day or 28 day back. It should be started from 5th day of the period and the tablet should be taken Daily at the same time without fail. It is a good method for most women under 35 years of age, who don't smoke and are educated. A woman having high blood pressure, diabetes, shortness of breath, chest pain, swelling or pain in leg, severe headache, liver disease, irregular bleeding, treatment for fits and a lump in breast should not take pills.

A woman taking the pill can have uncomfortable feelings like, nausea, vomiting and weight gain but she is releaved of menstrual cramps and excessive bleeding.

Injectable: The woman has to return for next injection every two or three months depending upon the brand of injection she is taking.

Implants: 'NORPLANT' is inserted on the inner side of left upper arm. One implant lasts for five years.

The follow-up has to be very meticulous and should be done every three months.

Non-Steroidal Contraceptives

Centcroman, 'Saheli' and 'centrone' are non-steroidal contraceptives.It has no hormonal activity and does not interfere with functions of other organs. It is marked as 30 mg. tablet which is to be started from 1st day of period. It is to be taken twice a week for first 3 months and then once a week. It can cause delay in period uptil 45 days. The chances of user failure is very high.

It should not be taken by a woman with recent history of jaundice, or liver disease, polyceptice ovarian disease, chronic cervicitis or cervical hyperplasia. In other words the drug requires supervision by a specialist.

Barrier Methods

Male: Condom, Nirodh: It is an effective, economical, disposable and practical method of birth control. It is most widely accepted world over as there are 19-25 million users. It does not require medical examination, supervision or follow-up and there are no side effects on the contrary it provides protection against STD and AIDS. It is supplied by the government and marketed also. If used properly with spermicidal jelly it is highly effective.

Female: Diaphragm, Dutch Cap & Cervical Cap: These are made of special rubber and are applied by the women to cover the mouth of uterus, thus preventing sperms to go up and meet the egg. They should be used with spermicidal jelly. These have a high failure rate as dislodgement can occur during the act. The size has to be decided by a specialist and it requires privacy to put it in besides it can predispose to infection if left for longer time or if removed earlier than 8 hours and can result in pregnancy.

Recently, Vaginal rings containing spermicide or progesterone are available to give protection for 30 days.

Female condom 'Femidom': This is also tried recently. It is made of soft thermoplastic polythene polycerethane sheath which loosely fits the lower canal and covers the outer organs.

Natural Methods

Withdrawal Method: In this the act of intercourse is interrupted before discharge and the discharge is done outside away from female organs. It has no contradictions but has a very high failure rate. Psycological tension to both partners can mar the spontaniety of the act.

Rhythm Method: The basic principal is to detect 'discharge of egg from ovary' and to avoid contact one week before and after it. If a lady menstruates every 28 days, the time of egg discharge is 14 + 2 days and unsafe period will be from 8th to 18th day.

Time of 'discharge of egg' can be calculated by temperature recording in the morning or by noting the changes in discharge from reproductive track. It has a very high failure rate.

Miscellaneous Methods

Douches, tablets or jelly to kill the sperms. It is not a practical method and has a very high failure rate. Besides it predisposes to infections as it removes the protective secretions of the genital tract.

Permanent Methods

These should be adopted by couples who have attained the desired family size. The age of the younger child should be more than 2 years and eldest child to be more than 5 years. These methods are 99 per cent effective but reversal is difficult.

Male Vasectomy

It is a surgical procedure that prevents the man's sperm from getting into his semen. The men's tube carrying sperms are cut and tied. It is a simple, safe, 99 per cent effective quick operative procedure. No follow up is required. Additional method 'Condoms' should be used in the first three months as sperms are stored beyond the cut end of the tube.

Now vasectomy is done even without a cut.

Female Tubal Ligation

This surgical procedure blocks the woman's fallopian tubes, so that egg and sperms cannot meet. A number of methods are prevalent like abdominal tubectomy done through a cut 'mini laprotomy' or with the help of a instrument 'Laproscope'. Tubectomy can also be done through 'Vaginal' the lower genital canal. It can be done just after periods or after childbirth or MTP.

16

INFERTILITY

Dr. Abhilasha Chaturvedi, D.G.O.

One of the reasons a couple consults a doctor is because they are not able to conceive. Here ultrasound has proven itself to be of tremendous use. It can give a picture of the internal organs, and it can also show the functioning of the ovaries.

1. All the organs of the lower abdomen can be seen well with ultrasound. A tumour of the uterus can be identified as a cause of infertility. A problem with the lining of the uterus can also be detected, especially with transvaginal (internal) sonography. However, it is not particularly useful in determining whether the tubes are open or blocked. For this, an X-ray of the uterus, or a diagnostic laproscopy are preferred.

2. On the other hand, sonography is almost routinely used to find out if the ovaries are producing eggs (ova) normally. In such patients, ultrasound is done every day, or sometimes on alternate days, to see the progress in the growth of the ovum—when does it achieve a mature size, and when does it rupture. The time of rupture is important as it is the best time for conception. This test is particularly useful in those women who have irregular periods, and those who are on treatment specifically to promote egg production. At the same time, the condition of the lining of the uterus is also assessed to see whether it is ready for a pregnancy. For patients who have to have artificial insemination (AI) or intra-uterine insemination (IUI) done, ultrasound will determine the best time for these procedures. In large centres, sonography via the internal route is also used to harvest several ova from the ovaries. These eggs can be injected with sperm by a special technique (a type of in-vitro fertilization or 'test-tube baby') and the embryo or early baby is then introduced into the uterus of the mother.

Pregnancy

Here also sonography has been of immense use to the doctor, because it does not harm the growing baby, unlike X-rays which can cause deformed babies. Another major advantage over other tests is that it can directly demonstrate the heartbeats and movements of the baby as they occur. The information provided by a good ultrasound examination during pregnancy helps the doctor in making decisions pertaining to the time and type of delivery, and any specific treatment the patient may require during the course of her pregnancy. There are several things the sonologist looks for during the scan.

1. How many babies are there? Usually there is one, but twins are often seen, and there may at times be three babies also. More than three can occur but are rare.

2. What is the position of the baby inside? In a normal pregnancy, the head is down and is the first part to come out, but the baby can have its breech end coming out first (medically upside down). Sometimes, the baby can be oblique or transverse, in which case a normal delivery may be impossible.

3. Is the baby alive? The heartbeats can be clearly seen by sonography, and the movements of the child are also seen. Heartbeats can be detected as early as one and a half months after the last period (2 weeks after the missed period).

4. Is the baby moving normally? The doctor is interested in knowing if the baby is moving enough, and if the type of movements are normal. This information helps the doctor to judge if the baby is having any problem inside the uterus, in which case an urgent delivery is required.

5. What is the correct age or size of the baby? In patients who are sure of the date of the last period, various measurements taken help to confirm if the baby is growing normally, or whether it is small or large for its time. In those who do not know their correct date, ultrasound will help in estimating the correct age of the baby, within a range of 1-3 weeks. The earlier the pregnancy, the more accurate is the estimated age. Towards the due date, the estimated age can be up to 3 weeks more or less than the actual age of the baby. This and the general condition of the baby have to be kept in mind while deciding when to deliver the baby.

6. What is the location of the placenta? If the placenta is present at or near the mouth of the uterus, the normal delivery passage is blocked, and so an operation may be required to get the baby out. Also, there is an increased chance of severe bleeding occurring from the vagina, which can be dangerous for the mother, and in such patients, an internal examination should not be done.

7. Is the amount of fluid around the baby normal? Knowing the amount of fluid around the baby helps the doctor decide the mode and time of delivery. If the baby is weak and the fluid is less, then it may be better for the baby to be delivered before its due date, as it may develop problems inside the mother. On the other hand, if the fluid is significantly less in the third to the sixth month, or much more than it should be, it may indicate that there is some major defect in the baby, and that the baby may not survive, or that it may require an immediate operation after birth to correct the defect. Again, this information is of use to the doctor in deciding the time, place, and mode of delivery.

8. Is there any abnormality of the baby? This is one of the major ways in which sonography helps the doctor. In patients who are detected to have severally abnormal babies who definitely will not be able to survive after birth (as when the head does not form, or the kidneys are defective), the parents may decide not to continue with the pregnancy at all. In others where the baby has a major but surgically correctable defect, with a good chance of a normal life later on, then the delivery can be performed at a hospital equipped to handle such babies and the medical or surgical problems associated with that abnormality. In those babies who are detected to have a major defect and whose quality of life is uncertain, the parents may opt for a normal delivery in preference over a caesarian operation. However, each individual patient is unique, and no general rules can be strictly adhered to in such circumstances.

Repeated Abortions or Bad Obstetric History

1. One of the causes of repeated abortions is premature opening of the mouth of the uterus. This can be corrected by putting a circular stitch at the mouth of the uterus before it has opened up fully. Ultrasonography can identify this dilatation of the mouth, and can aid in the diagnosis of this problem in mothers at risk.

2. Abnormal structure of the uterus (for example, a double or split uterus) can also cause abortions or premature delivery, because

there is less space than normal. Some of these patients can be treated by surgery. In others there is no cure since the problem is a congenital one, but knowing that the mother has this type of problem would alert the doctor and total bed rest can be advised in the second half of pregnancy, in order to prolong the duration of the pregnancy as far as possible.

3. Yet another cause of recurrent miscarriages is the presence of a growth in the uterus.The tumour diverts a part of the mother's blood intended for the baby to itself, and thus deprives the growing baby of much-needed blood and nutrients.

Other Problems

1. Lumps or masses in the abdomen can be of many types and can arise from any organ. Ultrasound can identify the nature of these lumps (whether they contain fluid or solid matter) and which organ are they attached to, if any. It can also evaluate the surrounding organs to see if the mass has any adverse effect on them.

2. Ovaries. : Tumours of the ovaries are a common cause of a lump in the abdomen. In the older age group, cancer is a likely possibility and although ultrasound cannot 100 per cent confirm or rule out cancer, it does give a clue to the likely diagnosis.

3. In women who have an intra-uterine contraceptive device (IUCD), the thread of an IUCD should normally be seen when the doctor does an internal examination. However, sometimes it cannot be seen. In these patients, the doctor cannot know if the IUCD has been passed out, or if it has penetrated through the uterus and is lying inside the abdominal cavity. An X-ray will show whether the device is inside the patient at all, and an ultrasound will show whether it is in the uterus or not.

4. There is an increasing incidence of ectopic pregnancies, or pregnancies which are not in the normal place (inside the uterus). The commonest of these is a tubal pregnancy, and an early diagnosis of condition is essential, because if the pregnancy ruptures (as it usually does after 6-8 weeks), it can lead to severe and life threatening internal bleeding. In such patients, an operation is necessary to remove the abnormal pregnancy. If the pregnancy is identified early enough, before it ruptures, it may be possible to save the tube from being blocked subsequently. However, it must

be kept in mind that an ectopic pregnancy can occur, and the ultrasound scan may not detect it and show a normal report.

Like all other investigations, ultrasound can be and is of immense use to the treating doctor, provided that all the relevant clinical information pertaining to the patient is given to the ultrasonologist, and that the result of the ultrasound scan is interpreted in correlation with the patient's problem.

Procreation is a basic instinct of every living creature. Although a few ultramodern couples are reluctant of taking additional responsibility of their children, even more couples at a subconscious level miss the joy of parenthood. Although they divert their unfulfilled desire of parenthood by involving themselves in other creative fields, their suppression of natural instinct may lead to frustrations and perversions in later life.

Apart from voluntary infertility, approximately 15 per cent of married couples fail to produce children, many of them can be treated by a scientific approach.

Causes

It may be 10 per cent in female or male or in both 20 per cent. But in a lot of cases the correct cause can be diagnosed and the others constitute a big group of idiopathic or unexplained infertility.

Impact of modern lifestyle on fertility status tends to be negative because usually the age of marriage is going up and in females the fertility declines sharply after the age of 28 years. The best age for child bearing is between 20-25 years.

The ambitious career oriented girls usually involve themselves too deeply in their professions. Their busy schedule may lead to infrequent sexual exposure and a very limited fertile period. When ovulation takes place she may not be covered by the sexual act. This may disturb their biological clock which has a very serious adverse effect on the hormonal system, so ovulation may be suspended. Crash dieting may lead to disorders like anorexia nervosa when even the menstruation stops due to poor nutrition and disturbance of the endocrino system.

Premarital sex is usually associated with unwanted pregnancy ending in abortions. This may lend to sexually transmitted diseases and also create pelvic inflammatory diseases and blockage of fallopian tubes.

Tobacco, alcohol and smoking also decrease the fertility.

Tight underwear and heavy jeans and synthetic clothes increases the scrotal temperature and causes autolysis of spermatozoa.

Late nights increase psychological stress. Excessive use of sex also influences 'gamtogenesis' (formation of sex cells) in both sexes. Atmospheric pollution by local carbon monoxide and insecticides also leads to infertility and abortions.

Infections like small pox, mumps, etc., may lead to testicular damage in males. Varicosity of testicular veins in common cause of male infertility.

Luckily this disorder can be corrected by a minor surgical procedure. Undescended testis, if not corrected in time, can permanently damage the testicles. Treatment depends on the extent of the disease.

Causes in Females

Commonest cause in India is genital tuberculosis.

Endometrios is common among western countries. This disease is cropping up in the affluent class in India practising family planning.

There is excruciating pain during menses, irregularity of menses and menorrhaoea. Treatment depends on the extent of the disease and is the job of a gynaecologist.

When to Consult a Gynaecologist for Infertility

Apart from the above mentioned problems, one should consult a gynaecologist after one year of unprotected sexual life after marriage. In case the women is above 30 years, the couple should wait for only six months.

Instructions

All the records of past and present treatment should be well maintained.

Obesity and general diseases of the hormonal glands such as thyroid disorders, diabetes, abnormal hirsutism of the body are some of the other causes of infertility and one should always consult a gynaecologist.

Investigations

Semen examination of husband should be done. Z Post coital

test of the vaginal and cervical discharge within 12 hours of coitus will show viability of the spermatozoa.

Thorough clinical examination is needed. Endometrial biopsy should be done premenstrual or within 12 hours of menses and the most modern method is sending out ovulation by Follicular Monitoring. In this USG is done through the vagina. By serial USG if we find ovulation, insemination should be done. Hormonal assays should be done in specific situations but these are very expensive.

Treatment

This depends on treating the cause if found. In unexplained sterility, it is advisable to have a holiday to avoid the stress and set the biological clock. One can improve sexual life by providing privacy and relaxation particularly at a cool atmospheric temperature which is beneficial and may cure infertility.

Patency of the fallopian tubes cleared by either USG or X-ray with dye injected into the uterus and laproscopy test is done after cessation of menses.

Avoid using lubricants during coitus and vaginal douching.

Cause of Male Infertility

Men refuse to have semen test and much less, treatment of oligospermia and azoospermia (less sperms and no sperm). To improve spermatogenesis there are medical and other therapies.

Semen wash and intra-uterine insementics may be done. Latest techniques in obsolute azoospermia by taking syringeal aspiration have developed. Sperms are taken out directly from testical and female ova are taken out and fertilized in a petridish or test tube baby.

Micromampulation spermatozoan outside the body single sperm is injected into ovum which has been taken out from the abdomen and fertilized.

Artificial Insemination

This method is easy to perform successful and simple, economical and successful ratio is very high but it has to be repeated. Generally semen is taken to inject into uterus from the husband if semen test is normal or with the consent of the couple semen is taken from the semen bank and injected in the uterus.

Female treatment depends on the causes of infertility. Anti Tuberculosis hormonal diseases treatment.

In case of no ovulation cycle, there are drugs to induce ovulation. The drugs have to be administered under thorough USG monitoring.

In case of tubular block, repair of the tube may be done by micro-surgery laser, etc., but the success rate is very low. If it is irrepairable the patient can go in for test tube baby, an expensive job, and it should be done by an expert.

Surrogate Motherhood

When ovaries are functioning despite an absent uterus, ovum is fertilised outside the body by the husband's semen and inserted into the surrogate mother. There may be emotional or legal problems. Ovum donation is another interesting development in the treatment of infertility. Now there are facilities for fertilized ova and sperm. There are banks for the same.

In spite of such dramatic techniques of treating infertility adoption has its value, particularly baby of some relation.

Sterility is one of the great source of stress—psychological, physical, financial and can cause depression.

Advice to Young Girls

Do not plan family very late in life. Do not sacrifice your natural instinct for your career.

Do not neglect menstrual irregularity and system disorder.

Avoid extra physical and mental strain. Avoid addiction to drugs, smoking, doing excess dieting or MTPs (abortions).

17

CARE OF THE NEWBORN BABY

Dr Abha Malik, M.D.

A newborn baby born between 37 and 41 weeks of gestation is termed as a full-term baby.

Feeding the baby— As soon as the baby and his mother are ready for each other, the baby must be put to the breast.

The watery 'colostrum' must not be discarded as it is rich in minerals and vitamins and protects the baby against diseases like polio and measles.

The mother should demand feed her baby, i.e., whenever the baby wants a feed, give to him, even at night.

Prelacteal feeds and extra water are not needed by a breast fed baby. A good burp dispels the swallowed air and prevents abdominal distension and vomiting.

2. Keep the baby with the mother so that the baby is warm and comfortable.

3. Babies cord should be kept dry and not covered by cotton or bandages. A soothing oil massage may be done.

Keep the baby clean by sponging him daily till the cord falls off. Then you can bathe him every day with a gentle soap. A mild powder can then be used, making sure it does not enter the baby's eyes.

The age old practice of *kajal* and oil in the ears must be discarded.

4. Normally babies pass urine and 'meconium' the dark tarry stools, within 24 hours of birth.

Problems in a Newborn baby that need not worry the parents

1. Skin
    - (a) Milia or white spots on the nostrils and face.
    - (b) Red spots in the white of the eyes-subconjunctival haemorrage.
    - (c) Blue Mongolian spots on the buttocks, reddish areas in the skin anywhere over the body.
    - (d) Peeling of the skin and vernix caseosa or cheasy material on the skin at birth.
2. Epithelial Pearls on the hard palate and tip of penis.
3. Hormonal Changes
    - (a) Breast enlargement (swollen breasts).
    - (b) A little vaginal bleeding in females during 3rd to 7th day of life.
    - (c) White vaginal discharge.
4. Deciduous teeth, if loose can be removed.
5. Physiological Jaundice of the newborn from 3rd to 7th day.
6. Caput succedaneum or the soft swelling on the head.

These conditions generally settle down as time goes by.

When to go to your Paediatrician Immediately

1. Jaundice on 1st day of life.
2. Excessive vaginal bleeding.
3. Blood stained vomit and refusal to take the feed.
4. Urine and motion not passed within 24 hours.
5. Coughing and frothing while feeding and respiratory distress.
6. Rolling upward of eyes, sudden jerky movements of limbs or a vacant stare, especially after a difficult labour.
7. Excessive crying.
8. Haemorrhagic spots forming all over the body.
9. Large pustules over the skin creases and rest of the body.

18

IMMUNIZATION

Dr. Abha Malik, M.D.

Prevention is better than cure and immunization is essential for all babies to protect them against common childhood diseases.

BCG and OPV in the first month of life should be given.

Three shots of Triple Antigen and OPV doses should be given from 6th week onwards to protect against Diphtheria, Pertusis or Whooping Cough, Tetanus and Poliomyelitis. An interval of 4-8 weeks between the injections may be maintained. Slight fever for 48 hours and local hardness may be experienced that will subside in a few days.

The 5th OPV can be administered with the Measles vaccine between the age of 9-12 months.

Injection MMR Vaccine between 15-18 months will protect against Measles, Mumps and Rubella or German Measles.

Boosters of Triple Antigen and OPV are given at 1½ - 2 years and again at 4½ - 5 years of age. If this 2nd Booster dose is delayed then Injection DT (Dual Antigen) can be given in place of Triple Antigen.

Latest vaccines recommended are:

1. Engerix B Vaccine against Hepatitis B—a serious type of Jaundice.

2. Typhoid vaccine— Oral and injection both are available.

3. Meningitis vaccine— depending on its availability.

Injection Tet vac should be repeated every 3-4 years during childhood.

For RH negative mothers with RH positive babies, it is very important for mothers to have their Immunoglobulin injection within 2-3 days of delivery.

19

PREMATURE BABIES

Dr. Abha Malik, M.D.

A baby born before 37 weeks of pregnancy, irrespective of its weight, is called a premature baby.

Premature babies must be kept warm and comfortable. Their mothers may eat light, nutritious food which is not very greasy or spicy, and should breast feed their babies. Demand feeding may be followed initially. When fed, the babies must be awake so that they can suck and swallow slowly.

Burping the babies in between and after a feed is important to prevent regurgitation. Totally breast fed babies do not need water in the first few months of life. Iron supplements may be given to them to prevent anaemia.

Their motion must not be watery and urine should be passed at regular intervals.

Kajal, oil in the ears, rough massaging and handling should be avoided. To prevent infection, visitors must be restricted from entering the room of the mother.

20

BREAST FEEDING

Dr. Abha Malik, M.D.

Breast feeding is nature's invaluable gift for a newborn baby. As soon as the baby and mother are ready for each other, after delivery, breast milk or colostrum must be offered to the baby. If, however, the baby remains hungry then supplement mother's milk with top feeds may be given. Use a cup and spoon to feed the baby, avoid bottle feeding to prevent loose motions, and colic, commonly associated with bottle fed babies. Breast milk is rich in minerals, nutrients, and has calories as required by the baby. Infections like poliomylitis and measles. Indigestion, loose motions, colic, vomiting, and abdominal colic are prevented in breast fed babies due to antibodies in the milk. Mother's milk is rich in Vitamin A which is good for eyes and prevents recuent infections.

The mother can give demand feed. The uterus also contracts dire to breast feeding and she feels satisfied suckling her newborn baby. Quick pregnancies are also delayed. Breast feeding is economical and time is saved as there is no bottle washing and sterilization to be done. The risk of infection, breast and ovarion cancer, is also greatly reduced in the mother.

Always start on the breast the baby finished with last time. He or she should usually have 10 to 20 minutes on each breast, but there is no need to time him. He will stop feeding when he is full. Halfway through the feed unlatch him and put him to the other breast. Do not worry if he takes different lengths of time over each feed. If he only takes a little milk at one feed he will take more the next. Do not press the breast while the baby is feeding. This only blocks the milk ducts.

To remove the baby from your breast when changing breasts, either slip your finger between the areola and the baby's lips or gently pull down his chin. When the baby has had enough he may continue sucking gently until it falls asleep.

Hand-expressing Milk

You may sometimes need to express your milk by hand. Place the index finger and thumb on the areola, and gently squeeze and push back towards the breastbone in the same movement. Do not squeeze the nipple.

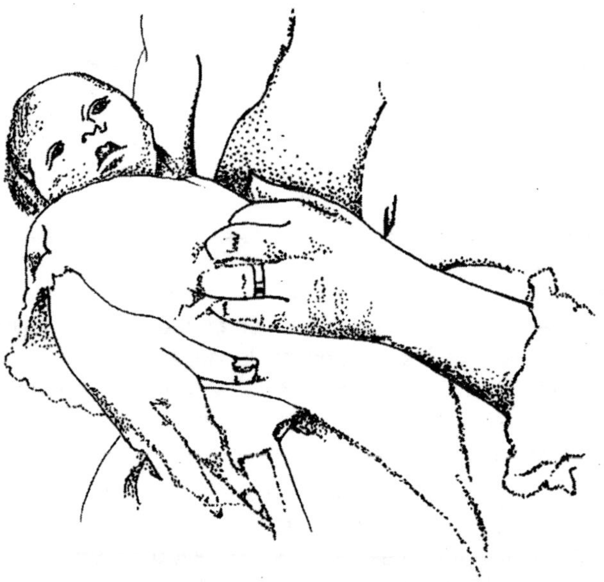

I Cradle the baby so that his mouth is level with the nipple. Support his head with your elbow or forearm. Gently stroke his cheek nearest the nipple. This lets him know that the breast is near.

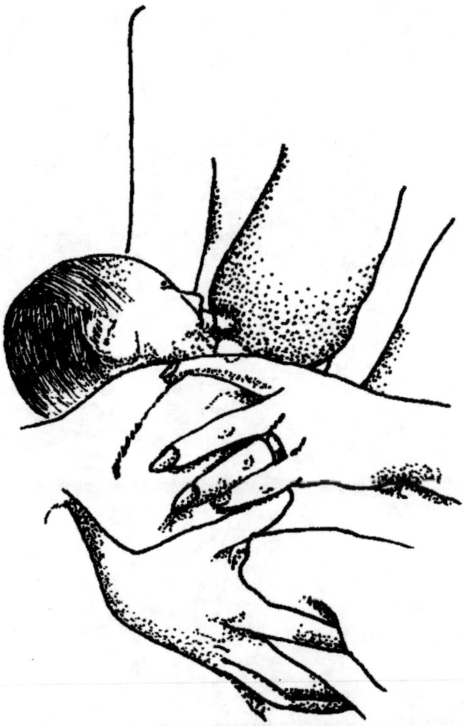

The baby will turn his head towards the breast, purse his lips and touch the nipple. He will then take the nipple and areola in his mouth and start sucking. Do not let the baby suck on the end of the nipple. He will get no milk because his sucking closes the openings in the nipple, and you will get sore nipples. Make sure that the nipple and areola are both in his mouth.

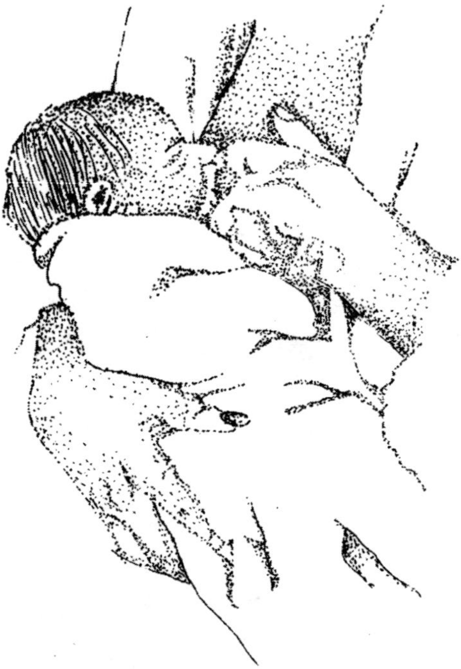

If the baby seems to have difficulty in 'latching on', hold the breast between finger and forefinger at the edge of the areola. Gently press and guide the nipple into his mouth. It may be necessary to press nearer to the nipple if the nipples are very flat. If the breast is too swollen for the baby to grasp the nipple it sometimes helps to express a little milk before putting him to the breast.

21

FEVER IN CHILDREN

Dr Abha Malik, M.D.

Fever is a common problem which troubles the sick child and worries his anxious parents.

How to Take Temperature of Children

Normal variation of temperature between 98° to 99°F is alright in children which is measured by a clinical thermometer. In small children axilla or groin reading is done. On adding 1 to the reading will give us the accurate body temperature. In older children temperature is taken subligually and is useful. In very sick children a rectal reading can be used.

What to do

Keep your child amidst cool environment when he has high fever.

Offer sips of cool water to prevent dehydration. Do not cover him with a blanket or quilt which will not help in reducing the fever.

If the temperature is above 100°F use an antipyretic advised by the doctor.

Do Not Use Aspirin

Cool compresses of the forehead, palms and soles with tap water helps in reducing the temperature.

Short duration fever may be due to a sore throat, common cold and cough which would be of viral origin. Mild gastroenteritis could give rise to temperature and when it subsides, the child does not look very ill. However if the fever is of a long duration the child may appear really ill. He has behavioural changes, irritable, and looses appetite. He may vomit due to high temperature. Such fevers may be typhoidal or due to bacterial infections of the liver or urinary tract. It could be Malaria, respiratory infection or even meningitis.

The child needs prompt pathological investigations and treatment.

Contact your doctor if your child has high fever and any of these conditions:

(i) irritable behaviour

(ii) convulsions

(iii) rash all over the body

(iv) severe cold and coughs, vomiting or diarrhoea.

Never ignore a fever in a child.

22

GASTROENTERITIS IN CHILDREN

Dr Vatsala Samant

Gastroenteritis is common in childhood and may be associated with dehydration. A child may loose much water and electrolytes during an attack of vomiting and diarrhoea. If the child has frequent attacks it may become dehydrated and malnourished.

To look for signs of dehydration—

(a) irritable or very sick child

(b) anterior fontenalle depressed

(c) swollen eyes

(d) dry mouth and tongue

(e) reduced quantity of urine

(f) skin thickness is reduced

(g) very thirsty or refusing milk and water.

Causes of Gastroenteritis

In babies below the age of six months and in younger children the Rota Virus is the commonest cause of gastroenteritis especially during winters. In the older age groups diarrhoea may be of bacterial origin as the children often eat food cooked outside their homes. Cholera, typhoid, E coli shigella are common causative organisms. Worms, Giardia and Amoebic infections also lead to diarrhoea.

Symptoms

In infections due to Rota Virus, early vomiting is followed by severe diarrhoea. In cholera the rice water type of large stools are present along with vomiting. The child becomes severely dehydrated. In Giardia or Amoebic infections, blood and mucus are present in the stools along with griping pain preceding a loose motion.

Prevention of Vomiting and Diarrhoea

(1) Wash hands before eating

(2) Eat covered food not contaminated by dust and files

(3) Wash fruits and vegetables before eating

(4) Drink filtered or boiled water as needed

(5) Cut nails regularly

(6) Wear shoes or chappal

(7) Bathe regularly in clean water.

What to do at Home in Case of Vomiting or Diarrhoea

(1) ORT Oral Lehydration Therapy to be started immediately. Sips of fluids like water with sugar and salt should be given every five minutes. In case of vomiting, wait for about 10 minutes and start giving fluids after every five minutes. Light tea, clear dal or vegetable soups, coconut water or whey, rice water, fresh lime or apple juice can be used to rehydrate the child.

(2) Maintain nutrition with *khichdi,* curd, banana, stewed apples, lightly buttered toast will keep the weakness associated with diarrhoea. Binding agents are not used nowadays as they only prolong the infections infectious period in the gut. If the vomiting or diarrhoea still persists and the child starts getting dehydrated, contact the doctor immediately.

23

SOME CHILDHOOD DEFORMITIES

Dr Vatsala Samant

Hare Lip and Cleft Palette

This is a deformity of the lip and palette present at birth. Development of the lips is twofold—a part coming from the left side and another part coming from the right side and joining in the middle to form the lip. Due to some genetic cause the two sides do not join and the result is hare lip as seen in a bunny. These abnormalities are usually obvious. Cleft palete can be seen only on the roof of the mouth when the child is crying. The tendency may run in families. The result of this abnormality is that there is difficulty in sucking from the breast or bottle and the baby has to be spoon fed right from birth.

Cause is not known but some medicine taken during the three or four months of pregnancy may cause this deformity. Ruebella infection of the pregnant mother may be one of the causes.

Treatment

This can be rectified by plastic surgery. These operations are successful. Operation at three months age has been very successful.

Anencephaly

This is an abnormality in which the major part of the brain of a foetus fails to develop. The bones at the back of the head are also partly or completely missing. Death occurs on birth. It is hereditary. It can be diagnosed by USG in unborn.

Treatment for Cleft Palette

Plastic surgery when the child is three months old. These operations are successful in many cases but may have to be done two to three times. I have delivered two or three such cases and the deformity has been completely cured by plastic surgery.

Mental Retardation

Mental retardation or MR may be defined as subaverage general intelligence manifesting during early developmental period. The child has diminished learning capacity and does not adjust socially.

Intelligence comprises of perception, memory, recognition, reasoning, verbal facility, and moter competiece. Intelligence tests are devised to measure different parameters of intelligence in the different age group. The degree of mental handicap is designated Mild, Moderate and Profound. The terms educable and trainable are used for mild and moderate handicaps. The severe and profoundly handicapped are called Custodial. However all levels are educable and trainable to some extent.

MR is due to inter play of several biomedical, socio-cultural, and psychological factors and it is difficult to incriminate a single cause.

Causes

(1) metabolic, (2) chromosonal, (3) developmental defects such as micraphaly, (4) use of teratogenic drugs in the first three months of pregnancy, Rubella, radium therapy during pregnancy.

Predisposing factors

Low socio-economic status which exposes to environmental factors, such as an inadequate nutrition of the mother, as well the child, poor prenatal and intranatal care, lack of immunization, delayed treatment of infection, like meningitis, etc.

Low birth weight child is subjected to adverse genetic or prenatal environmental influences which may result in brain damage. Consanguinity of parents is associated with high incidence of genetically transmitted mental handicaps. Mongolism is caused by advanced maternal age use of Ultra Sonography test may be done to detect Mongolism. Associated defects of the musculoskeletal system, vision, speech and hearing defects are often found in mental handicaps.

How to diagnose MR to know family developmental history complete physical examination should be done. Examination of fundus of the eyes, I.Q., assessment should be done when the child is in optimal condition, not hungry, tired or sick. During pregnancy in cases where prenatal diagnosis suspects defect in amniotic fluid test may be done.

Risk of Occurance and Recurrence

In a study when two mentally retarded parents had offsprings, 14 per cent had normal intelligence but when only one parent was mentally handicapped 27 per cent of the offsprings were normal.

Prevention of MR

Genetic counselling, chances of metabolic disorders with recessive inheritance are high in consanguineous marriages. The parents should be informed about the chances of birth of a similarly affected baby of a sibling is due to metabolic cause. Mother over the age of 35 should be told about increased risk.

Vaccination of girls with Rubella should be encouraged. During pregnancy teratogenic drugs, hormones, iodines, antithyroid drugs should be avoided. Mothers should be protected from contact with patients suffering from viral diseases.

Neonatal infections especially of the nervous system should be diagnosed early and treated promptly.

Managements

Parents should be seen together. The diagnosis of the child be fully explained to them emphasizing the abilities of the child and not only the disabilities. Parents feelings and the home situation should be discussed. Physically the M R child needs the same care as any other child. If any disease is present it should be treated.

Psychologically such children need warmth, love and appreciation as well as discipline. Normal criticism and high appreciation with short-term of good objective, structuring of learning activities. Unnecessary harsh criticism results in withdrawal and hostile reactions. Institutionalization should be avoided. Day care centres, schools, vocational training centres, workshops are useful. Classes should be taken to educate mothers and families in caring for the handicapped in trying to develop their potential to the maximum in the effort to make them as independent as possible.

24

CONGENITAL MALFORMATIONS

Dr Vatsala Samant

Every organ in the body may not develop in a normal way with the result a variety of malformations may result in newborns. Malformations of the brain such as Anannechaphaly Hydrocephalus and spina bifida account for about half the cases. There is no doubt that the presence of an abnormal gene in the female or male germ cell before fertilization is a frequent cause. It is well-known that defects such as hare lip and haemophilia are often inherited.

Causes

Environmental Influences

Embryologists have produced practically every deformity known in man by light variation in the environment of the developing embryo. This suggests that influence of environment is the causation of congenital abnormalities.

Deficiency of Vit A

Experiments in cows who were fed on Vitamin A deficient diet during pregnancy produced a litter with various eye defects. Eye defective pigs were fed Vit A diet during their pregnancy and they did not produce eye defective litter. Whether these experiments have any bearing on the causation of congenital malformation is not known.

Foetal anoxia

Lack of enough oxygen (Foetal Anoxia) which is due to maternal heart disease placenta previa or in would be mothers staying in the hills at high altitude where there is less oxygen may be responsible for congenital malformation such as anencephaly, hydrocephalus spina bifida, etc.

Irradiation Exposure

Experiments in lower animals have shown that irradiation in early pregnancy either by radium or X-ray leads to abortion and various abnormalities if pregnancy continues. In the human pregnant female, short exposure necessary for diagnostic purposes do not cause any ill effect.

Infectious Disease

A Rubella or German measle is a contagious disease and is a cause of abnormalities. This communicable disease is spreading in India due to increased travelling from abroad. It is very common in Australia. It is well-known that Rubella is responsible for many malformations particularly congenital cataract. In view of this risk when German measles has been contracted in first four months of pregnancy theraputic abortion is fully justified. There was a case of Rubella, a woman was in her fourth month of pregnancy. Her brother-in-law caught the infection in the swimming pool and he gave it to his sister-in-law. She had fever and rashes and it was diagnosed as a case of Rubella. She had to undergo an abortion.

Prevention of Rubella: The most hopeful method at present available seems to be active immunization of female or adolescents so that they will not contact the disease in adult life.

Diabetes

Pregnancy in diabetic patients have a high incidence of congenital abnormalities. A patient had three or four still births with hydrocephaluse diabetes which was not detected. During her next pregnancy her severe diabetes was treated with high doses of insulin. She had a ceasarian section. She had a 19 pound baby which is characteristic of a diabetic.

Endocrine Influences

This may cause abnormalities in the development of the male and female organs of reproduction.

A question is often asked by parents of congenetically defective child about the prognosis of future pregnancies. Murphy from his studies states that in families already possessing a malformed child, the frequency of subsequent defective offspring was about 1.29 per cent comparable with 47 per 10,000 in the general population which is 25 times greater. When two defective children are born in a family the second defective child is likely to appear later on rather than immediately.

Mongolism

It is generally believed that the fault lies in the germ cell. Mongols have been born to mothers who had been subjected to therapautic irradiation during pregnancy. When a mother is over forty years of age, the probability that a mother will have a Mongol child is more. After the age of 35 years there is a chance of having a Mongol child. Fathers age has no influence in this. Most Mongols are in the lower grade mental deficiency and their appearance is characteristic. The palpable opening slope is downwards and inward hands are broad and the index finger is short. Tongue is often large and fissured and it protrudes. Mongol children are affectionator pelent calm, excellent mimics and may learn to sing. They become prematurely senile, 40 percent of Mongols die in first five years due to congenital heart disease which is frequently associated. They are liable to have pulmonary tuberculosis, only a few reach the age of 50 years. Treatment in such cases is of no avail.

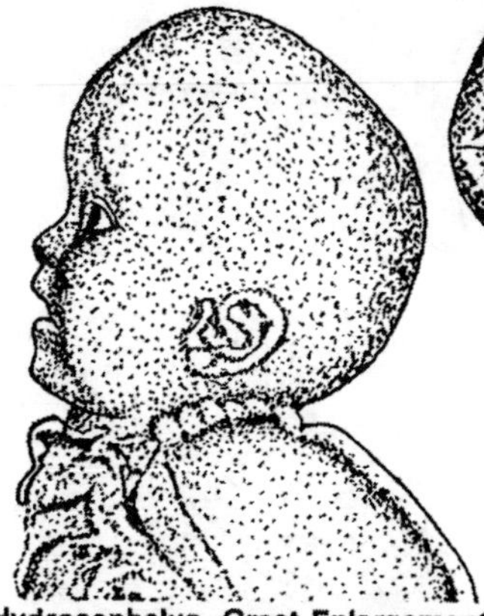

Hydrocephalus, Great Enlargement of Head, Making the face look Disproportionately Small

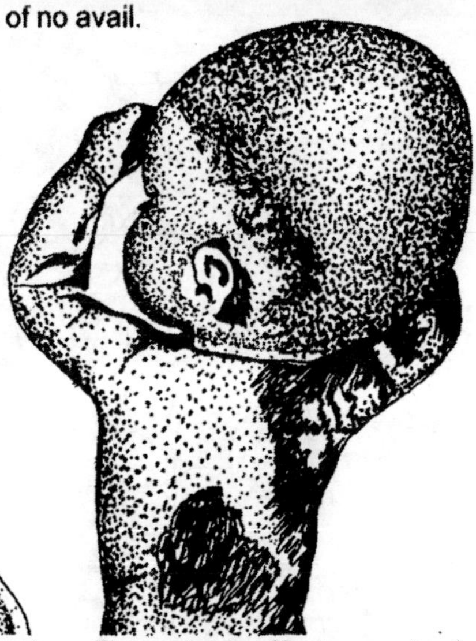

Thoracolumbar Meningomyelocele Arnold-Chiari defect and Intrauterine Hydrocephalus

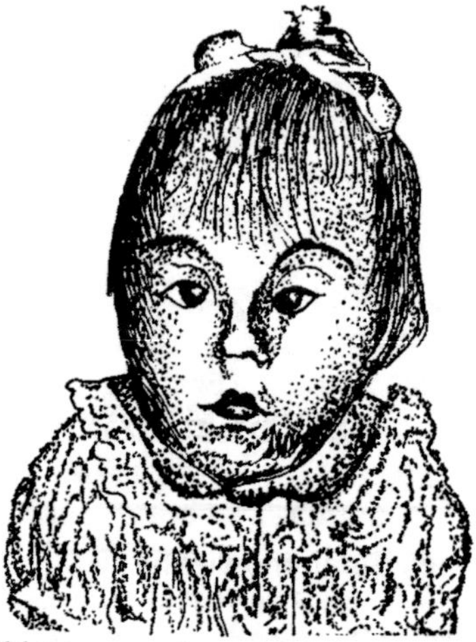

Typical facial appearance of young child with Down's syndrome

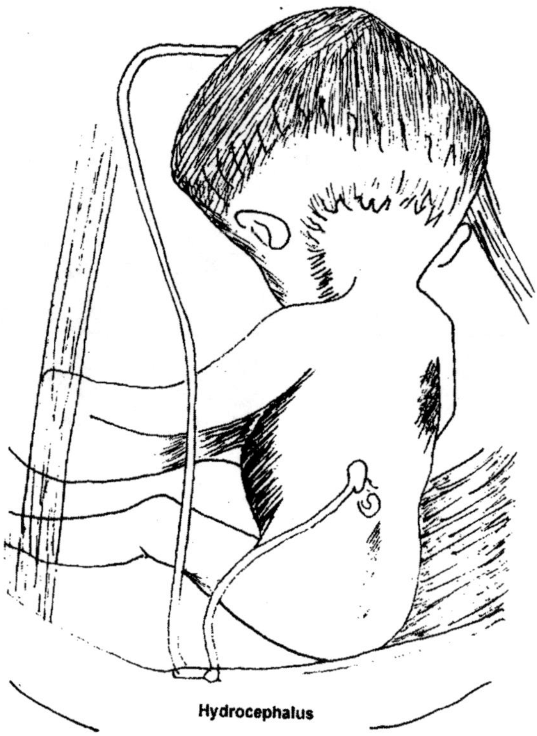

Hydrocephalus

25

DYSLEXIA

Dr Vatsala Samant

What is dyslexia? It is a learning disability, which selectively affects a child's ability to read and write.

In 1970, scientists began to suspect that people with dyslexia have some fundamental problems with their vision or hearing. Studies have since then suggested that victims have something amiss in the central cortex (brain), an important part of the brain responsible for thought and language. It is an area of tissue, which affects hearing by acting as a relay station for auditory signals. Genetic abnormalities are the cause in 90 per cent of the cases. Brain damage (after the person has learnt to read) due to high fever, trauma or head injury accounts for the other 10 per cent.

Symptoms

A tendency to confuse "up" with "down", "left" with "right", "saw" with "was", reading without comprehension and having trouble with arithmetic. These symptoms may be found in young children but if the symptoms linger on after the child is 7 years old then it is possible that the child is dyslexic. The need for careful observation and identification of the problem is essential. If not recognized and treated in time and the teacher calling the child "stupid" causes an emotional upheaval, which the child is unable to fathom leads to the child dropping out of school.

Of course there are some specific learning disabilities and when they are obvious, coping with them is simple. But sometimes this disability is left to be discovered till it is identified and dyslexia is one of them. After all it is essentially a language communication disease.

Dyslexia is more common in boys. Einstein, it is said, was dyslexic and did badly in school. Dyslexia cannot be cured or prevented but things are changing. Dr Suniti Sodhi since 1967 has opened learning centres giving an individual approach to specific needs. Many big cities have also adopted the concept and thus with specialized help the dyslexia has an excellent chance of coping with this problem and can go on to bring his intelligence and special talents for service of society.

Parents should get professional help to cope up with a dyslexic child.

26

AGEING

Dr. Vatsala Samant

Old age is the period when one has gone through the stages of childhood, youth, middle age and thus has reached the last stage. There are lot of bodily and mental changes which take place as we sail through life. With old age comes the degeneration of our cells accompanying which are the likely diseases or fear of diseases.

There is fear of high blood pressure, heart disease and cancer. Retirement from jobs, fear of disease and insecurity creates a vaccum leading to depression insomnia or sleeplessness and the thought any time you had to go on your final journey leaving behind your near and dear ones and everything you have earned through hard work.

It is not only the global population which has increased but the population of the aged has increased tremendously. Life span of an Indian has increased. This increase has led to many problems. Let us consider these problems. Due to urbanisation living conditions, joint family system is no more.

Aged people who used to rule the family have lost their authority which is difficult to swallow. There is feeling of insecurity and loneliness and a wide generation gap along with physical and mental disabilities, so on soforth makes the life of aged a problem to themselves and to their relatives. Philanthropic organizations, particularly Christians and Parsees have Homes for the aged. Homes have not solved the problem.

During one's old age when life comes to a standstill, one must develop hobbies and live with nature. Taking to religious activities is a very good way of staying peaceful throughout the day, at one with God. For the socially mobile people, social work is a very good and satisfying avenue which makes one feel contructive and worthwhile other hobbies may be: gardening, visiting places, looking after grandchildren, writing, music, etc.

Alzheimers Disease

Alzheimers disease or AD is the most devastating of all diseases because it attacks the very essence of our human nature, our ability to, remember, think and reason clearly. About 10 per cent people are affected over the age of 65. AD is caused by neuron disfunction and death in specific brain region, is responsible for cognitive function.

Symptoms

The first symptom of AD is the gradual onset of short-term memory loss, difficulty in remembering names, recent events, conversation, misplaced items, appointments, and repeating comments or conversation. Though it should be emphasized that mild memory difficulties occur commonly in older adults and the above mentioned symptoms can be present even in the absence of the disease. The age associated memory impairment does not interfere with social or occupational activities. Patients with AD exhibit inability to learn new skills. Personality and behaviour changes are present, remote memory past events are retained early in the disease. In the mid stage of AD patients become disoriented have worsening of languages, short and long-term memory loss. They loose ability to calculate, may, become suspicious, have delusions, hallucinations and other behavioural changes.

In the later stages, there is complete loss of judgement, little meaningful speech. Later on there is loss of mobility. They become pathetic and withdrawn, unable to recognize loved ones. There is incontinence of urine and require 24 hours care. The average span of life from diagnosis to death is approximately eight years.

The major barrier to progress in AD is a lack of understanding of the causes and how these causes bring about changes in the brain. It is likely that the causes are genetic, environmental, increasing age, head injuries. A drug Ibuprofen may slow the progress of AD and may prevent it altogether. AD symptoms controlling the disease may be simple, as lowering blood pressure, exercising, quitting smoking but there is no cure as such.

Senile Vaginitis

Perium or private part is full of bacteria harbouring near the anus, inter and the urethra. It is estrogen, an ovarian hormone that keeps the vaginal health. During menopause and old age estrogen production is stopped and the vagina becomes vulnerable to bacterial attack, an infection and causes vaginal itching of the vulva due to vaginal discharge, which is worse at night making one sleepless and miserable.

Treatment

Treatment is genital hygiene, but no antiseptic lotion should be used. Aeration of the part, i.e., exposing it to air and mild sunshine is also useful. One must wear soft cotton clothes which should not be very tight. To keep the vulva dry do not use a rough towel but use a soft piece of cloth. Application of mild cream and in some cases even HRT (Hormonal Replacement Treatment), a very mild dose of estrogen after consulting the doctor.

27

GLAUCOMA

Dr. Vatsala Samant

Glaucoma is a symptomatic condition and not a disease. There is increased intraoccular pressure. There are two types of glaucoma—primary and secondary.

Secondary glaucoma is due to inflammation of the eyes and many other factors such as lens injury. There is dimness of the vision and halos. There can be an acute pain with vomiting and dimness of vision. The chronic phase which if not treated gradually passes into blindness. Acute form occurs preferentially in women in their fifties of an excitable nature. Primary glaucoma occurs in either sex, over sixty years of age, who are of no specific psychological pattern. Both can lead to blindness. The disease is insidious and not noticed until the vision of one eye is almost lost and the other seriously impaired when it may be discovered.

What is glaucoma?

There is pressure in the Intraoccular region when the intra-occular tension is increased the disease is known as glaucoma.

There are two varieties of glaucoma :

(a) ***Primary-*** when it occurs without anticedent disease.

(b) ***Secondary-*** when it follows as a result of some existing disease.

Primary glaucoma occurs under two forms:

1. Inflamatory or congestive.

2. Non-inflamatory or non-congestive known as simple inflamatory is either acute or chronic.

Symptom- In all cases of glaucoma there is disnunition of vision and fogginess and cornea looks cloudy. In acute cases they may be slight swelling, pupils, are dilated and sluggish in reaction to light. The tension in the eye is increased.

Causes are insomnia, too much worry, insufficient food, glaucoma is a disease of advanced age. Both eyes are affected -

Treatment cases of glaucoma should be treated with all care .

Consult a doctor particularly on aged people. Doctor will decide about operation gridectomy or selerotomy may be done to reduce the tension, glaucoma can lead to blindness.

General Treatment : All cases of glaucoma should not suffer from constipation.

They should take light diet, green vegetables, milk and fruits are helpful. Do not take too much of tea or coffee, no drink they should avoid late nights and sleep care. Any eye error should be corrected, morning exercise is good and they should have proper rest to the body and mind.

Medically, some eye drops advised by an opthalmalogist should be used once or twice a day a conslipation should be corrected wife blizxksy or mild laxative, Harda Murahha and guland is good. Then should be hot bathing if eyes by vapour with *Tulsi* leaf.

Nature cure vapour bath thrice a day, warm water tub bath, light yoga asanas.

28

CATARACT

Dr. Vatsala Samant

The lens in the eye is a biconvex transparent mass which becomes opaque and is known as cataract. Acquired cataract is due to the degeneration of the lens fibres. Many factors lead to this degeneration. The most common is ageing. Senile cataract is rare in persons under 50 years of age except in diabetic patients, but is almost universal in some degrees in persons over 70. It is common both in men and women and is usually bilateral. It may develop in one eye and then in the other. There is a genetic influence in its incidence and in hereditory cases, it may appear at an early age and also in successive generations. The rate of development of senile cataract varies greatly, sometimes taking many years.

There is a variety of cataract known as congenital particularly in children affected by Rubella, and mongolism or Downs Syndrome. There was a patient who was expecting her first baby. She was quite young and yet she had cataract in both the eyes and so also her younger sister. A baby was born and the child had bilateral cataract.

Symptoms

The early complaint is that of seeing spots before the eyes, doubling, or trebling of the objects seen with the eye. There may be a change on colour values.

Treatment

No medicin treatment by drugs or otherwise have been known to have any significant effect in inducing disappearance of cataract once opacities have developed. In all cases, careful examination should be done to exclude any specific or constitutional cause of the disease. Once the cataract has been matured the only effective treatment is operation. There should not be any restrain on using the eyes, in uncomplicated cataract. The patient should be assisted by some one. Dark glasses are usually of great comfort when worn outdoor. Eyes should be examined every six months once the cataract development has started. Even in senile cataract the opacities may remain localized for years without any serious disability. In every case diabetes should be ruled out.

Cataract

In cataract the pupil instead of being dark beems light grey or some other colour due to the opacity of the focussing lens of the eye. When the lens becomes opaque, the rays of light from different objects do not pass through the lens and the vision is lowered the patient becomes more or less blind.

Cataract has been observed for many thousands of years. There are various theories about causations if cataract, primary cause being pressure on the eyeball. The memory of imperfect sight produces a shein on the outside muscles of the eyeball which is accompanied by a contracetion of these muscles and cataract is produced.

The obvious symptom if cataract is opacity of the lens.

Senile cataract is common and seen after forty-fifty heridity may be the cause.

Traumatic cataract is due to any injury at any age one of my corosion while playing with small cane got hurt in one of his eye and developed cataract and lost his vision.

Congenital Cataract is due to faulty development I had a patient with congenital cataract who delivered a child with congenital cataract general disease such as diabetis, other general disease can cause cataract symplin, opacity of the lens, dimness in vision and cloudness, when central feels difficulty in sking light and seen better in dimlight.

Treatment are causes of cataract must be educated to relax their mind, good food habits, avardane of some kind and drinking, vapour chash, walks on device in lawn is helpful.

Certain if eye drop of Japan has proved in many cases if early stages of cataract.

Optical mlologist should be consulted and in Senile cataract if the lens opacity is mature surgery is the answer. These days long stay in the hospital is not needed, operation is done with the help of lesser & a lens is fitted if patient walkout for the 24 hours before operation diabeties, anemia & other disease have to be ruled out.

29

VARICOSE VEINS

Dr. Vatsala Samant

The twisted elongated, unsightly veins that pop out just beneath the skin surface are varicose veins other sights are oesphagus, scroturm and anus. A malfunction in the mechanics of blood circulation or an inherited weakness of vein wall causes varicose veins. Normally valves in the veins of the legs keep circulating blood from drainy back down once it has desired oxygen to the tissues of the limb. If the valves fail blood flows downward forms pools and eventually cause veins near the surface to become swollen and contracted. Prolonged periods of standing and lack of exercise contribute the condition. Amongst woman hormonal changes and pressure on pelvic veins during pregnancy may lead to very veins.

Women should set with their feet proped up with legs raised above chest level. Avoid obesity. Standing for a long time, exercising legs by walks.

A cold compress utilise essential oils is helpful. Longstanding varicose veins can cause eczema of the feet which can become septic and painful in such cases surgery is beneficial.

Tuberculosis

T.B. is increasing as a result of many factors, HIV infection, increasing survival of elderly, worsening social deprivation (infected as children and now reactivating and increasing drug resistance). Pulmonary infection is about 75 per cent and extrapulmonary 25 per cent. In some disease progresses with a development of miliary meningeal, tuberculosis, Bone, Kidneys and miliary T.B. is a severe infection often diagnosed later. Patient has fever, tiredness, swelling, etc., shows fine millet sead appearances through looks the lungs. T.B. is a notifiable disease.

Prevention: The last protection against T.B. is the efficient diagnosis statement of people with active lesion household and other similarly close contacts of patients should be screened by T.B. skin test and X-ray. The test is used to assess whether a person has acquired T.B. following exposure and is useful in person not immunised with B.C.G.

B.C.G. gives 80 per cent protection for 20 years.

T.B. lymphadenitis - enlargement of lump glands most learned of certical (H.cap) & mediastinal, axillary and inguisial. The lumph holes are painless, molale and can cause abscess. They should be removed by surgery and sent for Hystopathology.

Abdominal T.B.

T.B. Peritonilise, Asertis, palpable mases if malted omentum and intestine caccum is sometimes affected and there is narrowing, distorture and shortining and one can feel a lump third side below the liver.

An accurate diagnosis is the first in any treatment plan and there is always a danger of self-diagnosis.

Homeremetic

1. Ginger: Though a food and spices has been used medically for centuries. It is used for treating cold, nausea. Ginger oil massage can alleviate skinal and girnt problem. Ginger tea is good for stomach ache and digestion.

2. Garlic: Early in this century garlic was used to treat T.B. and it is an antibiotic thus a great potential for treating cardiovascular conditions and it can reduce cholesterol and high blood pressure. It is a safe herbal remedy. Some people are allergie to gastic and in some it may cause stomach unless and anaema.

3. Anamon is carminative releasing gas from stomach and intestines.

4. Basil is carminative and when brewed in tea it is supposed to aid digestive and may be helpful in relieving stomach cramps, vomiting and constipation.

5. Anisen is used coughs syrup and lozenges.

6. Liquorice in cough and chills it has expectorant, antiallergic and antiinflamatory properties. Long term and excessive use can produce headaches lethargy, 'High Blood Pressure'.

30

RHEUMATOID ARTHRITIS

Dr. Vatsala Samant

Rheumatoid arthritis is a progressive slowly destructive swelling of the joints particularly affecting the joints of hands and feet. Later on it spreads to wrists, knees, shoulders, elbows and ankles. There are repeated attacks. The age group is between 25-55. More than twice as many women as men are affected.

Symptoms

1. Swollen joints, stiffness, pain in the affected joints.
2. Red shiny skin.
3. Limited movements.
4. Sometimes fever, weight loss and feeling of ill-health. It can last for many years.

Blood tests can confirm the diagnosis, X-ray of the joint will show the severity of the disease. Prevention is not possible. Outlook is poor, cases of rheumatid arthritis run a long course of alternate attacks and semi-remissions and eventually cause destruction and deformity of the affected joints.

31

OSTEOARTHRITIS

Dr. Vatsala Samant

Osteoarthritis basically is excessive ageing. Larger joints are usually affected. Sometimes hands and feet can also be affected. Obesity leads to a higher incidence. Obese persons have 61 per cent of osteoarthritis of the knee joint as compared to 20 per cent in thin persons. Onset is slow and earliest symptom is stiffness of the joint which is experienced after rest and may disappear on movement. Gradually pain becomes severe, joints get swollen, and there is a continuous gnawing pain all the time. Walking becomes difficult and during night moving in bed is painful. X-ray can confirms this. Osteoarthrits can be more adequately controlled and is amenable to treatment in the early stages. Avoidance of injury is very important. The affected joint should be rigidly protected from the slightest injury and excessive movements of the joint should be prevented. Weight reduction also helps. Physiotherapy is of great help. Diathermy sittings, massage, hot fomentations, give a great relief. Few passive and active exercises have to be done regularly.

32

OSTEOPOROSIS

Dr. Vatsala Samant

Osteoporosis is a major age related problem. It affects the skeleton of our body. There are about 203 bones in our body, a huge solid mass that supports our body. Osteoporosis is a condition characterized by a reduced amount of bone mass which leads to diminished physical strength and susceptibility to fracture. There are many causes of osteoporosis but the most common and by far the most important is due to the decrease in the amount of bone mass that occurs after the menopause though it starts at menopause in women and continues progressively with age. Men do not undergo an abrupt fall in their sex hormones as do the women and also men have a greater skeletal mass than women and women outlive men and thus osteoporosis is more common in women than in men. Due to osteoporosis there is a crush fracture syndrome which occurs between 55 and 65 years of age and on the other hand there is a hip fracture syndrome occurring after 15 years.

Post-menopausal bone loss causes no symptom but there is a risk of fractures of any bone, particularly of wrist, vertebrae and hip. Osteoporosis is therefore a significant cause of morbidity and even mortality and so represents a major problem of health care.

The two major risk factors are the low bone mass in women particularly thin women and magnitude of the subsequent bone loss. Bone loss is determined by genetic and also environmental factors.

Bone loss is also determined by menopausal age, and is mainly due to deficiency of ovarian hormone or sex hormone and also by a very low calcium intake and unhealthy lifestyle. Advanced age, early menopause, removal or irradiation of ovaries, low body weight in comparison to height, increased liability to fall, suboptimal diet, low calcium intakes, coffee, tobacco, alcohol, certain drugs and immobility are the causes of osteoporosis. The skeletal system of an osteoporosis patient can be compared to a fragile vase. With ageing, liability to fall not only increases but protective reflexes become progressively impaired. When an elderly person complains of back pain or when a woman is admitted with hip fracture person not due to an accident, one can think that it may be due to osteoporosis. X-ray and developed technology for detecting bone mass will confirm this.

Recently, advanced technology has contributed to the rapidly increasing knowledge of the pathogenisis, prevention and treatment of osteoporosis. Balanced diet, reasonable intake of calcium, protein, carbohydrates, fat; exercise, abstinence of coffee, tobacco, alcohol and H.R.T. (Hormone Replacement Therapy). Small doses of ovarian can increase bone mass and prevent fractures. Bone loss starts the onset of menopause. Bone loss can be due to certain diseases or drugs particularly cortico-steroids though age is a major factor. Defects in the diet and lifestyle should be corrected. Certain drugs are being tested for prevention of osteoporosis as an alternative to hormone treatment.

To summarize the methods of preventing osteoporosis, menopausal women should be encouraged to have adequate intake of calcium 500 mg, Alfa Vit. D, sunlight therapy and daily exercise. When a woman has experienced several osteoporotic fractures of spine and hip, possibilities of cure by medicine are limited to symptomatic aids and chronic care of the patient is the only remedy. It is very important to eliminate environmental factors which may have a negative effect on the skeleton. All the hazards that increase the risk of fall should be eliminated. There is a great risk of falling when bathrooms are wet. One should remain physically active and do simple exercise.

Table Showing Calcium Content of Food

Food	*Calcium in gms*
Cottage cheese	100
Egg	40
Ice-cream	75
Skimmed milk	130
Swiss cheese	950

Yogurt	120
Sardines	420
Shrimp	120
Beans	100
Lettuce	100
Onion	35
Orange	40
Potato	5
Resins	50
Spinach	100
Bread white	50
Bread white whole	70
Bread brown	100

33

STAYING HEALTHY THE NATURAL WAY

Dr. Vatsala Samant

Healing is a natural process common to all life wounds heal by themselves in people just as in animals and plants. If we want to faster healing and promote health we should pay attention to the ways nature and learn to encourage our body's own inate mechanism of self-repair. Our defence system to fight invasion of frequencies, trarema, chemical weapons, is better than any country's defence system.

Alopathic therapy, discovery of effective drugs antibiotics, development of immunisation, modern surgical operation is a golden age in science and technology can do away with poverty illiteracy, hange and disease. At the same time science and technology though solving the problems of health has created many problems for example, modern medicine has succeded in reducing sickness, premature death due to infectious diseases now medicine has to deal with more difficult types of illness particularly in an ageing population which is growing at a rapid rate such and are a pray to cancer, heart disease, mental illness. And naturally public is disillusioned and many of the ancient systems of treatment which were under celepse are coming back in light and attracting number of patient.

High Tech. High cost modern medicine with all the technoligical methods has been very expensive that many people cannot afford. Not only the high tech medicine is expensive it can also be dangerous and frequently harmful did as adverse drug reactions which can because permanent disability or death. During may house surgeonship one of our wardboy had an injury and naturally antitetnic serium was injected which caused instant death. Even then there are solid achievements doctors can treat victims of trauma more effectively acute infections like Pneumonia that killed people in the past Preventing of death in medical and surgical emergencies greatest achievement is preventing former fatal complication of childbirths, anirades of reconstructive surgery, such a giving new hip or knee forms destroyed by injury or illness, greatest achievement is immunisation, preventing, major killers polio, deptheria, Telanus we cannot replace modern medium by alternative therapy conditions which are treated by modern medicine, the first requirement for taking more responsibility for your health. When a problem demands immediate interventions by scientific medical methods, in short emphasis should be on self-care and personal responsibility for willingness.

Despite these achievements there are other alternative methods based on natural traditions healing practises, such as acupuncture, herbal medicins since handed down from mother to daughter.

Health Care Means Rolling

1. Role of nutrition 2. Value of mind power 3. Your role in your own care

1. Role of nutrition: In the medical curriculum very little importance is given to diet therapy, except for the fact that empasis was on special diets for hospitalised ailing patients. But now it is generally accepted that high fat, low calorie specially these high in meat and low in vegetables predispose to cancer of colon, breast and uterus. Vitamins were supposed to benefits in preventing processor diseases, like scurvy, but recent research has shown Processor of Vita Beta carotone has cancer inhibiting effects against cancer of breast, cervix and Vitamin B, lowers cholestrol, Vit E is used in the treatment fibuestic disease of the breast and same is the case with minerals used therapatially, garlie one of the most prominent healing hurt in the folk tradition of many cultures, does have antibiotic properties, garlic is supposed to lower high blood pressure. I spent my childhood in a village type of town Bassein and I remember my grandmother used to bandage a boil on fect using hot gastic and it used to heal the boil.

2. Value of Mind Power: Health care means, mental emotional, spiritual aspects of health and not just physical body, after all mind is as important as liver or spleen, etc., in our body. Therapies like hypnosis and visualisation which are supposed to change physical conditions though purely mental intervention, these therapies are safe cheaper than in vasive procedures, there are cases in which pain killers did not work a cure but, keeping the mind in good moods and laughing have had beneficial effect and the diseases have been cured, after all body has a head and the head should come first. And so there is laughing therapy for sick people in and out of hospitals.

3. Your Role in your own care: Your body your own care the best thing is staying well rather than look for cancer and yourself taking the whole responsibility for your health, it will not only save your money, no risk if medical toxicity and help you to avoid further health problems. Be an active participant in your well being than a passive recepient if health care. Understand that your body has a remarkable power of healing and repair, natural medicine begins and ends with that simple truth and it is your job to make intelligent choices of methods to activate and enhance those powers.

34

PREGNANCY AND ITS HAZARDS

Dr. Vatsala Samant

Every woman desires to become a mother. Motherhood satisfies her emotional needs. It gives satisfaction and a kind of euphoria to nurture a child, nurse the baby, protect it, teach it and make the child into a fine citizen—naturally the mother is proud. After all, the hand that rocks the cradle, rules the world.

Nature has ordained that the female of every species, including mankind, is the one to propagate the species. This is her main natural function, and so information about pregnancy and the hazards associated with it should be known to every woman.

Pregnancy is the result of the meeting of a tiny spermatozoa travelling through the Fallopian tube, with the ovum, from the ovary. What is called a Zygote, or fertilized ovum, is formed in the tube, and it must move all the way to the uterus, where it is welcomed, embedded and nurtured. Sometimes due to obstruction in the tube, it cannot reach the uterus and tries to grow in the tube which is thin walled and cannot stand the strain and there is a serious problem. This condition is known as Ectopic pregnancy.

Proper care is essential. Midwifery, or obstetrics is the science that deals with the prevention and treatment of complications, to ensure a healthy mother and a healthy child.

Some of the possible complications are as follows:

1. Ectopic Pregnancy: During the first two or three weeks of pregnancy the lodging of the zygote in the tube may cause this to rupture, causing internal bleeding in the abdomen, pain, shock and collapse if not treated. If not operated on immediately, it may even prove fatal.

2. Morning Sickness: 50 per cent of all women suffer from morning sickness. If there is continuous and severe vomiting, however, it can lead to dehydration, weakness and acidosis, unless hospitalization and intravenous glucose infusion is provided. As a rule, morning sickness stops at three months of pregnancy.

3. Abortion: This is the expulsion of the pregnancy before it reaches maturity. In 20 per cent of women, a pregnancy ends in abortion. There are various causes. Symptoms are vaginal bleeding, pain, almost like labour pain and sometimes shock. The best remedy is to consult a doctor who will decide to allow the pregnancy to continue or not.

4. Toxemia of Pregnancy: But if caught early, it can be cured completely.

5. Bleeding: The most dangerous is bleeding from the placenta. The placenta is the structure which feeds the foetus, gives oxygen and takes away waste products. Normally it is attached to the upper part of the uterus, but sometimes it is implanted in the lower, thinner part, near the cervical opening. There are a few contractions during the last months and this may cause separation of the placenta and antepartum (or before delivery) bleeding. It is painless; the patient may just find herself soaked in blood while asleep. The bleeding can be severe and even fatal if not properly handled. Toxemia may also cause separation of the placenta and painful bleeding.

The discovery of ultrasound sonography has been very useful in finding the site of the placenta so that precautions can be taken.

Post-Partum Haemorrhage (PPH) is bleeding after the birth of a child either before or after delivery of the placenta. Bleeding can be very severe and even uncontrollable, in which case removal of the uterus by operation is necessary. There can even be bleeding later, on up to about 40 days.

Pregnancy definitely causes strain on the kidney's. This can lead to high blood pressure, albumin in the urine and swelling of the body. If not diagnosed and treated in the early stages, it may lead to convulsions, coma, foetal death, and may even prove fatal.

6. Malpresentation: Normally the foetus lies head down, but sometimes it stays topsy turvy or even cross-ways, making delivery difficult. This can cause rupture of the uterus and even death, particularly among the rural population though modern techniques can be used to manage even this complication in hospital.

7. Infection: A delivery room has to be clean, aseptic, and the doctors and others masked and dressed in sterilised clothes. The greatest boon we now have fighting infection are antibiotics.

8. Injury to the Reproductive Organs: The tubes are injured in ectopic pregnancy. Injury to the cervix, vagina, perinium and even bladder are possible, and even rupture of the uterus in mishandled cases.

Thus, we can see that pregnancy can take its toll in the form of maternal death or disability. Maternal mortality is still unfortunately high in India, while in the developed countries it has been minimized to almost nil. Proper and balanced diet for the mother to prevent anaemia, prenatal care, checking of the blood pressure and weight gain, regular examination, blood tests and ultrasound when necessary, aseptic conditions for delivery and proper care has done a lot of good.

Knowledge of all this is also necessary. Along with the education of women, particularly classes on motherhood should be made compulsory in girls' schools.

35

OPERATIVE PROCEDURES IN OBSTETRICS AND GYNAECOLOGY

Dr. Manjula Pande, M.S.

Minor Operations

Endometrial Biopsy

This means taking out a small piece of the inner lining of the uterine cavity and subjecting it to pathological examination for diagnostic purposes—a very important and useful procedure in cases of infertility.

Dilatation and Curettage

Dilatation is the widening of the cervical opening (mouth of the uterus) which normally is closed so tightly as to not even allow the tip of small finger to negotiate through it. After this the next procedure is curettage of the uterine cavity, meaning scrapping of the content therein with moderate force. The contents removed by curettage are subjected to biopsy, thus establishing the diagnosis of various uterine diseases like uterine tuberculosis, malignancy, incomplete abortion and disorders relating to abnormal menses.

Curettage, sometimes, is done as a part in cases of abnormal and protracted menstrual flow and when patient is aborting.

Almost same procedure of dilatation and curettage is emplicit to terminate a pregnancy what commonly is known as MTP.

Major Operations

Caessarian Section

This operation is done to remove the baby from the mother's womb after opening the abdominal cavity and then the uterus. The exact procedure involves opening lower part segment of the uterus as it is easier to open, heals, better and bleeds less. There are many reasons when this operation is needed. Sometimes to save the life of baby and sometimes mother.

The operation is needed when the baby is big and the mother's passage is narrow or baby lying horizontally across the womb so that it simply cannot be delivered normally. Sometimes placenta is on top of the opening of the uterus obstructing the passage of the baby and causing massive bleeding. Sometimes the labour pains are abnormal and the mouth of the uterus fails to open or the labour proceeding towards normal delivery does not progress beyond a certain stage. Since the baby gets stuck in the mother's passage which again becomes a life threatening situation for both the baby as well as the mother, an operation is done.

It is a wrong feeling that once caessarian— always a caessarian. The passage of the mother having previous normal deliveries may need an operation and a mother who has had caessarian previously may have a normal delivery. A point of caution here is that if a mother has had two caessarians should have third delivery also by caessarian operation. This patient simply cannot be allowed to bear pains as the uterine scar may give way causing the uterus to rupture taking lives of mother and baby. A third caessarian has also to be accompanied by sterilisation for the same reasons.

Tubectomy

It means removal of the fallopian tubes. This procedure presently implies removal of a portion of tubes for the purpose of permanent sterilisation.

Hysterectomy

Originating from 'Hystero' which means uterus, 'ectomy' meaning removal so it is the removal of the uterus from the body cavity. This operation is required for the tumours of the uterus, excessive bleeding during menses which has not responded to medical treatment and cancer of the uterus. This operation is sometimes performed by the vaginal route when uterus descends down and comes to lie below the genital opening.

Laproscopy

This means making a small buttonhole near the naval and putting a telescope through it thus visualizing different organs inside the abdomen. This procedure is used for performing tubectomy, removing small tumours of the uterus, small cysts of the ovary and helps in the diagnosis of infertility. The advantage of laproscopy is its simplicity and short stay in the hospital.

36

ULTRASOUND

Dr. Madhu Mittal, M.D.

There are a variety of tests available to the gynaecologist to determine what may be wrong with a patient. One of the simplest is the ultrasound examination. There are other simple tests also, like the PAP smear, and post-coital test, but they give limited information and are used in specific instances. On the other hand, ultrasound or sonography gives a good picture of the uterus and surrounding organs, with no injections or X-rays required.

The ultrasound machine has a small probe which is moved over the patient's skin. Very high frequency sound waves are then passed through the patient, and the returning echoes are analysed by the machine to give a picture of the internal organs. This test is absolutely painless and harmless. All that is necessary for examination of the lower abdomen is a full urinary bladder. In some patients, a further internal (vaginal) ultrasound examination by a special probe may be required, and this also is painless and similar to the manual pelvic examination done by the doctor. This internal ultrasound examination is more accurate than the one done from the abdomen with a full bladder.

Ultrasound has also proved to be a boon to pregnant patients. Now the condition of the growing baby inside the uterus can be determined right from the time of confirmation of pregnancy till the delivery. Here also, a full bladder is required, but only in the first three months of the pregnancy. After that no preparation is necessary. In fact it helps if the patient has had a meal within an hour of the test except in cases where the gall bladder or liver also have to be examined.

Excessive or Irregular Bleeding

What does the doctor want to know in cases of excessive bleeding?

1. She would like to know whether there is any tumour in the uterus, how many there are, and where they are located—near the inner lining of the uterus, in its walls or towards the outer surface.

2. She would also want to know if the inner lining of the uterus is normal, or is there any abnormal thickening or growth in this region.

3. Is there any tissue left after an abortion, which is causing excessive bleeding?

4. What is the condition of the ovaries? Sometimes, tumours of the ovaries can cause irregular cycles. It also helps in deciding whether the ovaries also need to be removed in case of an operation to remove the uterus.

Scanty or Absent Menses

How does ultrasound help in patients of reduced or absent menses?

1. First of all, it can determine whether or not a uterus is present in a girl who has not started her monthly menstrual cycles. The size of the uterus can also be seen.

2. The ovaries can be well seen even in girls who have not started menstruation. If they are not identified, then they may be absent or small. Sometimes, swelling of the ovaries can result in irregular scanty menses. This can be detected, the ovarian size measured, and the response to treatment assessed, by sonography.

3. Is there a pregnancy which is causing absent menses? Often, after a delivery, the periods stop because the mother is feeding her child. In this circumstance, another pregnancy may occur of which the mother is not aware. Ultrasound can help confirm the presence of such a pregnancy and determine its age.

37

MATERNAL MORTALITY

Dr. Vatsala Samant

Health of the women has been the primary concern of all cultures, because the seeds of future generation develop in the womb of a woman. India has highest maternal mortality. Approximately 9500 mothers die in a year, that is, one mother every 4 minutes. Our mortality is about 50 times higher than in developed countries. This is due to poor prenatal care. Formerly reproductive health meant "Safe Motherhood" but now it covers a much wider field. It includes normal anatomical and functional development of genital track, regulation of fertility, healthy practices and enjoyable sexual life.

Another foremost task before us is the care of the adolescent girls. They are faced with several changes during this period—physical, physiological, psychological, and sexual. If they are not properly counselled at this stage lot of harm can result. They have to be made aware about risks of unsafe sex, genital hygiene, etc., Quite a large number of teenage girls become pregnant because of unprotected coitus and can be victims of STD. Boys and girls have opportunities to mingle in schools, picnics and during social functions. The risk of pregnancy has to be weighed against the risk of lowering moral standards. Adolescent girls must be told about hazards of pregnancy and their prevention. Fifteen per cent of pregnant women are adolescents and they account for a disproportionately high rate of maternal morbidity and mortality. Most pregnancies are unplanned and unwanted and have an impact on the physical, emotional, educational and economic status of girls who are between the age of 15 to 19 years.

We must make an effort to reduce maternal mortality in our country. This can be done by the schools, NGO'S, women organizations, etc., by making the young girls aware about all the aspects.

38

GENITAL HYGIENE

Dr. Vatsala Samant

There are several simple steps that can be taken to ensure that one's genital area remains healthy. When washing, avoid soap getting into the vagina. It may cause thrush to develop. Vagina is a self-cleansing organ and does not require antiseptics. Dettol lotion shoud not be used while washing the private parts. Only water should be used for this purpose. After a bowel action be sure to wash from front to back to reduce the risk of contamination. Consult the doctor if you have any vaginal discharge or vulva irritation.

Good personal hygiene is essential. It will prevent the spread of bacteria which are always there and cause infection of the genital track, i.e., vaginities and prarities. During pregnancy bath should be taken everyday.

39

VAGINAL DISCHARGE

Dr. Vatsala Samant

Discharge per vaginum is a very common complaint. Vulva and vagina are normally moistened by secretions of the glands in the cervix at the *introitus* or opening of the vagina. Women who are over anxious and suffering from the fear of venereal disease and cancer, exaggerate the symptom and so called complaints of discharge depends much on ideas, patients' observation and fastidiousness of the individual. Sometimes they complain of foul odour. Provided a reasonable standard of cleanliness is maintained, vulval odour is never apparent and it is more a disorder of the mind than of the body. The idea of odour usually arises from a misconception of some remark of an acquaintance and therefore becomes an obsession with the patient and is difficult to eradicate.

Normally there is always a slight discharge at the vulva and there is a change in the appearance and quality or quantity of discharge during the menstrual cycle. There is watery discharge after menses and then it becomes like the white of an egg which again becomes thin before menstruation. During pregnancy discharge is increased. In the newborn girl there can be discharge for one to ten days.

Puberty discharge is commonly seen in young girls during the few years preceding menses, and unless the fussy mother does not make the child introspective this is a temporary phenomenon which corrects itself in due course.

Pathological Discharge

Inflammation and infection of the genital track is due to injury or an inserted foreign body in vagina or uterus. A sudden onset of discharge means infection of the genital track. Growths and noncancerous lesion of the vagina or cervix causes blood stained and purulent discharge.

Cancer of the vagina and cervix causes a foul smelling, and blood stained discharge per vaginum and is a sign of advanced cases of cancer.

Pathological examination of the discharge—a film on glass slide can clinch the diagnosis of the disease.

Pruritis Vulvae

This means itching of the vulva. This is a symptom which is experienced by not less than ten per cent women who attend gynaecological clinic. It is troublesome at night when in bed and causes sleeplessness.

Causes

Skin of the vulva gets irritated by vaginal discharge due to infection causing scratching which then becomes ulcerative. Other causes are skin diseases such as scabies. It may be manifestation of allergy to soaps, bath salts, cosmetics and particularly hair removing substances. Similarly condoms used as a contraceptive can cause allergic pruritis. Pruritis can be a manifestation of marital disharmony and a protective mechanism of avoiding coitus.

Chronic skin diseases like leukoplakia or precursor of cancer can cause pruritis. The first and only symptom of diabetes particularly in older patients is prutitis vulva and leukoplakia.

There is one variety of vaginitis due to Trichomonas which is associated with itching.

It can be diagnosed by studying a vaginal smear and its treatment consists of taking pills by both the partners, husband and wife.

Treatment

Depends on the cause, if found, treatment is satisfactory and vice versa if the cause cannot be detected.

It is important to prevent scratching and ensure sleep by giving sedatives and cold cream application. The part should be kept clean, free from sweat by wearing loose and light clothing. Airing of the urea part by using fan three to four times a day helps in reducing the intensity of the scratching and also wiping the part with soft cloth after bathing and washing after urination instead of using a rough towel.

40

URINARY TRACK DISTURBANCE

Dr. Vatsala Samant

Anatomically urinary bladder is an organ situated next to the uterus or a pelvic organ and naturally urinary disturbance are very common in women.

Enuresis

Bed wetting is the rule in children. It continues for variable number of years and can persist in adolescents and adults. In children it is best not to worry or scold as there is a spontaneous cure.

Bed wetting in adults can be a manifestation of unhappiness, insecurity and nervous tension. Taking fluids 3 hours before relaxing and emptying the bladder every 3-4 hours helps to cure bed wetting in adults.

Incontinence of Urine

This is an uncontrollable escape of urine or feeling wet all the time. True continuous flow of urine is due to a fistula or opening of the bladder in the vagina. Fistula is caused by operation such as hysterectomy and by difficult and obstructed labour. Vulva gets sodden and is a very distressing condition. Treatment is repair of the fistula.

Sometimes, there is prolonged and neglected retention of urine due to various causes and overflow incontinence.

Urgency Incontinence

Patient has to run to the toilet to avoid an accident because if she is too late the bladder empties. This generally is a malady of old age.

Stress Incontinence: This is escape of urine while coughing, laughing, walking and in certain cases turning in bed. Generally manifestation amongst aged. Vulva becomes irritated and patient is lead to changing of under clothes or wearing a towel and life is a misery and she feels a social outcaste, avoids leaving the house and with nothing else to do munches food and becomes fat, which adds to her discomfort.

Retention of Urine

During pregnancy if the uterus is displaced behind, she is unable to pass urine, sometimes for more than 24 hours and suffers from pain and swelling in her abdomen. Immediate catheterisation and keeping the chatheter in the bladder for 2-3 days helps her to pass urine. Uterine position is corrected by changing her posture and exercise.

Very often a woman neglects to empty her bladder due to over work, playing cards or watching TV and there is retention with loss of bladder reflex. Hot sit baths relieve retention. Retention is also due to nervous diseases like paralysis and during puerperium particularly after forces delivery and abdominal operation. Big tumours of the uterus can cause retention of urine.

Frequency of micturition is a very common phenomenon during early months of pregnancy due to pressure of the growing uterus on the neighbouring organ or the pressure of the presenting part of the infant and also infection of the urinary tract.

UTI

Infection of the urinary track is very common amongst women. Female urethra is very short, and opens on the vulva which lodges many types of bacteria. Anything that lowers her natural resistance to fight the disease leads to infection. Particularly after childbirth, incidence of UTI is very common. Frequent catheterisation is also responsible for the infection. Fever, frequency and burning during urination are some of the symptoms. Urine should be examined for pus cells, etc., and treatment entrusted to the doctor.

There is what is known as Honeymoon Pyelitis which is due to the slight injury during the first coitus.

41

INFECTION

Dr. Vatsala Samant

The genital track has an opening to the abdominal cavity for which there is a natural defence system against infection. There can be a variation in the efficiency of the defence mechanism, particularly during childhood, after menopause, childbirth or abortion. Infection can affect any organ of the reproductive system.

Infection of Vulva

Some of the common sites are hair follicles and glands in the vulva. Infection of these give rise to boils. This is also a manifestation of diabetes. Infection in the vulva is common around the age of five years because vaginal resistance has not developed. Bacteria are transmitted by hand, clothing of the children or even an adult. Quite often it is due to a foreign body inserted in the vagina by the child, for example, sand or shreds of clothing. The child may complain of pain, dysuria and discharge. It may spread to the eyes and also to other parts. It is important to avoid the child becoming morbidly interested in the genetic organs, which happens if the mother is over anxious. During old age the defence mechanism weakens and there is what is known as senile vaginites.

Infection of Uterus

Infection of the uterus, etc., can occur after childbirth. Tubercular Bacelli invade the fallopian tubes and uterus from the adjoining intestines and peritoneum. Manifestations of the TB are loss of weight, amenorrhoea and sterility and it can be diagnosed by blood test and biopsy of the endomentruim. I remember a case of sterility for amenorrhea for three years. On investigation she was found to be suffering from Tuberculosis of the uterus. These days TB can be completely cured with anti-tubercular treatment for two years she conceived and gave birth to a child.

Sexually Transmitted Diseases (S.T.D.)

In olden days gonorrhea and syphilis were vastly prevalent. The discovery of penicillin has minimized the incidence, even then, these diseases are still prevalent because the organisms causing these infections have become resistant to the antibiotics used.

The most dreaded diseases belonging to the STD family, AIDS (Acquired Immunity Deficiency Syndrome) has cropped up.

Our immune system is essentially one of the defences against invaders. The basic need of the defence system is to identify the alien or foreigner—bacteria, fungus or virus.

Fungus or Virus

AIDS is infection by HIV virus. One of the immunological defence is a T Cell the most important link in fighting the illness. The HIV virus affects and infects T cell so the recognition of the invading virus as a foreigner is lost. As in the legend of the Trojan Horse inside which the Greek soldiers were smuggled into Troy, the viruses are transmitted by the infected T cells into the circulation of the blood. The entire immunity system collapses and AIDS patients die either of infection, or of cancer on account of the failure of the immunity systems to identify the foreigners. AIDS is a dreadful disease for which until now no recognized cure has been found.

Our immune system has been developed to function as a biologic democracy where the individual members such as White Blood Cells and bone marrow achieve this end of killing the invaders through an information network. As this system is disrupted, the body's war against the virus is lost. AIDS is transmitted by sexual intercourse and is more common amongst homosexuals. AIDS is given to an unborn child, through the mother's blood. It can also be transmitted by syringes, to the nurses and doctors attending the patient in the HIV infection. In Western countries blood is tested for HIV during the antenatal period and the same has started at most hospitals in India also.

Another source of infection is through blood transfusion by professional infected donors and that is why blood transfusing, a life saving remedy becomes a life taking tragedy. To avoid this risk it is better to take blood of a relation of the patient. But in India most relations are unprepared to donate blood.

Tumours of the Genital Organs

We do not know why the cells of the organs multiply, particularly those of the uterus and ovary. They multiply in a systematic way and do not invade adjacent organs. They are known as benign or innocent tumours or growths, and if the cells multiply and invade adjacent tissues, they are known as malignant or cancerous growths.

Fibromyoma of the Uterus

This is a growth of the uterine muscles. It varies in size, situation and in number. But it can be present in the uterus during pregnancy causing trouble. Generally it manifests itself between ages 30 to 50 but it can occur any time after puberty. Generally it appears in sterile women and there is a saying either you produce a foetus, or a fibroid. Symptoms depend on the size and situation of the tumours. There is menorrhagia or excessive bleeding, pain, lump in the abdomen, discharge from the vagina and urinary symptoms. Diagnosis is very easy by palpation, internal examination and confirmation with sonography. Treatment depends on age of the patient, parity, size and situation and number of tumours. In young patients removal of the tumour or tumours is practiced. If not so young and with a complete family, the uterus is removed by operating because they can recur if the uterus is not removed, thus having the danger of their becoming malignant.

Benign Ovarian Tumours

There are a variety of tumours arising from the ovary. Particularly in a young girl a teratoma contains bones, teeth, hair, etc., and is supposed to arise from ebryonic tissue which are left over. A palpation of lump in the abdomen and X-ray showing bone, etc., confirms the diagnosis. Treatment is operation and removal. There are other tumours, quite a number in variety. They are either cystic or solid and some have hormonal disturbances. They may be either feminizing or masculizing. They have the nasty habit of twisting not only once but several times and causing acute pain in abdomen, shock, fainting, etc., and the only way is to rush to a hospital where an emergency operation is done.

Cysts not causing any apparent symptoms if detected during the check up, should be removed because of the danger of malignant changes in every case of ovarian or uterus tumours.

42

LEUKOPLAKIA

Dr. Vatsala Samant

Leukoplakia is a chronic inflammatory condition of unknown origin that affects the vulva, causing pruritis vulvae.

Clinical Features

It generally appears in the post-menopausal age, only the surface skin of the vulva is affected. The extent varies with the severity of the disease. Itching is the chief and only symptom though there may be pain and soreness.

Vulva is swollen, reddened, excoriated and the surface dry. Lateron colour changes to white semi opaque. Then cracks, fissures and later on ulcers appear and at this stage leukoplakia is liable to become cancerous.

Treatment

Relieve the itching. Vitamin A is supposed to be helpful. If conservative treatment fails, excision of only the affected skin should be done. Unfortunately the disease is apt to recur in the healthy skin drawn to cover the raw area. As this is a precarious condition, biopsy should be done in every case of leukoplakia.

Kraurosis of the Vulva

This is a condition caused by the loss of oestrogen after menopause, affecting only the mucous membrane of the vulva.

Red spots, bad patches appear. And there is dypariunia due to shrinkage of the introitus. Very often the condition is symptomless. In two to three years spontaneous cure may occur. Kraurosis does not become cancerous.

Treatment

Oestrogen vaginal pessary.

43

CANCER OF THE REPRODUCTIVE SYSTEM

Dr. Vatsala Samant

What is Cancer?

The origin of human being is from a single cell made up of the nucleus, the protoplasm and the cell membrane. This fertilized ovum goes on dividing, and increasing in number to form various systems—nervous, alimentary, muscular, reproductive, etc. In short, human being consists of billions of cells.

Normal cells have the capacity to regenerate when damaged and worn out, but in a systematic style and within normal limits. In cancer due to some factors, this same cell acts in a mad way, forgets its domain, goes on dividing and goes beyond its boundaries and invades other parts of the body. This cell is called a malignant cell and thus cancer is developed.

Causes of Cancer

There are various theories, but none is very satisfactory.

It was believed that if the same part of the body was constantly involved in injury then cancer is caused. For example:

(i) Injury to the cervix due to too many childbirths.

(ii) Injury due to burn by the *kangri* or small coal pot used by the Kashmiris in winter causes cancer of the skin.

(iii) Chewing pan all the time, and cancer of cheek.

(iv) Smoking causes cancer of lungs.

Cancer is not caused by poisonous gases spread into air, water or food by industry. Recent theories have shown that these are not cancer causing factors. There are biological factors found in the cells of the body, and there is foul play among cancer causing agents, environment and genes.

Each person is born with various genetic susceptibilities; or weak spots in his genetic make-up. Some persons have genes that enable their bodies to detoxify or destroy carcinogen cells rapidly, whereas other persons are born with slow acting varieties of the same genes that cannot get rid of these carcinogens when exposed to large quantities.

Another theory is that there is an enzyme found in the liver and other tissues which metabolizes or burns carcinogens. This enzyme actively declines with age. Hence cancer seems to be a disease of the aged.

In short, we do not know the exact cause of cancer. Cancer can begin in any part of the body from head to toe and from childhood to old age and in both the sexes.

Cancer of the Reproductive System

The reproductive system of a woman is made up of the ovary, the fallopian tubes, body of the vagina, cervix, vagina, vulva and breast.

To begin with, cancer is a painless disease. Pain is the last symptom to appear when the disease is far advanced. A few warning signs and symptoms of cancer in women are:

(1) contact bleeding

(2) foul discharge from vagina

(3) unexplained loss of weight

(4) anaemia

(5) after menopause bleeding

(6) swelling of the abdomen

(7) hormonal disturbances

(8) lump in breast

(9) discharge from the nipple.

Contact Bleeding

Contact bleeding is bleeding during intercourse and can be the first and the most important sign of cancer of the cervix.

Foul Discharge from Vagina

From puberty to menopause and thereafter, there is always a little discharge from the vagina. This consists of secretions from the cervical glands and varies during the menstrual cycle. First it is watery, then it is like the white of an egg. It is never blood stained except a few hours before the start of menses. It is never foul smelling. If found otherwise, it is a very important sign of cancer of the cervix and vagina. Any ulcer on the vagina which is not healing, or growth on it, is the sign of cancer of the vulva.

Unexplained Loss of Weight

It is a sign of cancer but not necessarily always present and generally occurs late in the cancer disease.

Anaemia

Less blood in the body is also one of the later symptoms during cancer.

After Menopause Bleeding

Menopause is the stoppage of menses between 45-50 years. Bleeding after menopause is the first sign of cancer of the body of the uterus and is the only sign.

Enlargement of the Abdomen

A person can be affected at any time with cancer of the ovary, from early childhood, middle age or old age. The signs are enlargement of the abdomen and sometimes hormonal disturbances.

I would like to mention the case of a young female child of 3 years who had developed a malignant turmour of the ovary. The signs were onset of puberty: enlargement of the breast, starting of menses and enlargement of the abdomen. But, due to illiteracy and superstition, she was proclaimed an "Avtar of Devi" and people flocked for darshan with gifts. Needless to say, an operation was refused and I lost trace of the girl.

Lump in the Breast

Any lump in the breast or the armpit, may be the first and only sign of cancer of the breast. Blood stained discharge or purulent discharge from the nipple is another sign.

Consult a doctor if any of the above signs manifest. Remember cancer can be cured if diagnosed in the early stages.

Every woman after the age of 35 should get certain tests done. These are cancer detecting tests. For example:

(1) PAP Test — i.e., cervical and vaginal smear.

(2) Mamography—i.e., injecting air under the breast and taking an X-ray to detect a tumour.

(3) Blood Test—There are certain blood tests done in America for detection of cancer.

Treatment

I have already said that if detected early, cancer can be completely irradicated. Dr. V. Shanta, Director of the Cancer Institute of Madras, recalls that the early fight against cancer, particularly in children, would appear to improve, but in a few months they would come back with a relapse.

But now a treatment protocal has been devised which has encouraging results even among patients with advanced cancer. The new approach is tackling the disease with antibiotics, surgery, radiotherapy and chemotherapy, either intravenous or locally into the tumour, a technique that has been developed recently. The important thing to remember is that early detection is possible only through regular check-ups. While cures are possible even at later stages, at the earliest stages the success rate is by far the best. Do not wait for pain to occur. Visit your doctor at any of the above signs.

44

CANCER OF THE REPRODUCTIVE ORGANS

Dr. Vatsala Samant

Cervical Cancer

Uterus has two parts—body of the uterus and neck or cervix. Cervical cancer (CA) with the single exception of the breast is most common in women. The risk of developing CA of cervix is increased by early marriage, irrespective of child bearing. The disease shows a marked predilection for women who have borne one or two or more children and the risk increases with each additional confinement so that a woman who has had six or more children is twice as likely to develop CA as the woman who has had only one child. In women, aged 35 to 64 the probability of developing CA seems be 1 in 21000 in single women and 1 in 6500 in childless married women and 1 in 1500 in parous women (Malphand).

Clinical Features

Usual age is 40 to 55 but it can occur at any age. Cases have been recorded—in one a patient aged 7 months and in another 93 years, having CA. The risk rises until the age of 60, beyond which it shows a steady decline. Of the affected 95 per cent are parous women and only 5 per cent are non-parous.

Symptoms

Unfortunately there are no early symptoms. The first symptom usually is bleeding from the vagina particularly after coitus. It may be a mere drop or two and be absent for days. To begin with there may be vaginal discharge which later becomes foul smelling. There is frequency of micturition dysuria rectal disturbances. In advanced cases, bladder is involved in cancer extention to these organs and which results in urinary and rectal fistulae. Lateron there is weight loss, anaemia, fever, pain, loss of sleep. Death is due to excessive bleeding or coma.

Examination

Diagnosis is easy in advanced cases. By just bimanual pelvic examination one can feel a growth. The difficulty arises in early cases of CA of cervix. Bimanual examination can feel some irregularity of the cervix and there may be blood on finger. There are various tests to detect vulnerable areas of the cervix.

Pap Test: A smear is taken with a spatula from the CX and studied to find out if there are any cancerous cells in the smear.

Surface Biopsy: A small piece of CX is taken and studded under microscope.

Treatment

(a) Surgery, (b) Radiotherapy, (c) Combination of both.

Advice

Examination of the cervix bimanually and speculam should be done of every patient and a PAP smear is a must for every woman after the age of 35 years. CA of cervix is a curable disease if detected early. I have treated cases of early CA CX by surgery and irradiation and followed them for 10 years with good response. The lesson lies that CA CX is a curable disease if detected early. Early detection is entirely in the patients hand to consult a doctor as early as possible. CA CX can be prevented by avoiding early marriages and having too many children.

Carcinoma of the Body of the Uterus

The greatest incidence is from 50 to 60 years of age and is rare before 40 years. It is always post-menopausal. 30 to 50 per cent are nulliparous women (no children) and if it occurs in parous women only in those who have had 1 or 2 children.

Symptoms

Women having excessive bleeding at menopause are three times more vulnerable to develop CA CX than the average women.

Bleeding from the vagina is the first sign and a slight Leucorrhea or discharge from the vagina may precede bleeding by several months. Foul smelling discharge is late in appearing. Pain is rare and is late and is due to extension of the CA. Bimanual examination shows uterus to be either normal or atrophic or even enlarged.

Diagnosis age is over 40 years.

Post-menopausal Bleeding

Diagnostic currettage can confirm the diagnosis. I had a case who was given irradiation to stop mennorragia. After she had bleeding from vagina D and C was done which showed it to be a case of uterine cancer. She had radical hystrectomy done and she is alright for the last five years.

Treatment is radical hysterectomy and radiotherapy.

Primary Cancer of the Ovary

These tumours are often silent until enlargement occurs. There may be gastro intestinal symptoms present years before abdominal

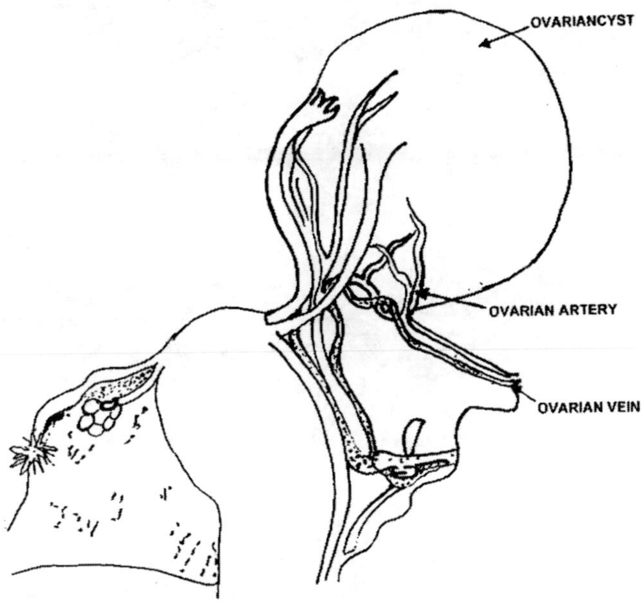

Structures of Ovarian Pedicle

swelling. Nausea, vomiting, loss of weight, pelvic pain and dyspnea is there. Cancer of the ovary does not occur before the age of 49 years. Any and every tumour of the ovary has to be examined for malignancy because even benign tumours can become malignant.

Treatment is surgery, radiotherapy and chemotherapy but the prognosis is bad because there is no early diagnosis, I know a case of a woman who was quite healthy and active. One day she

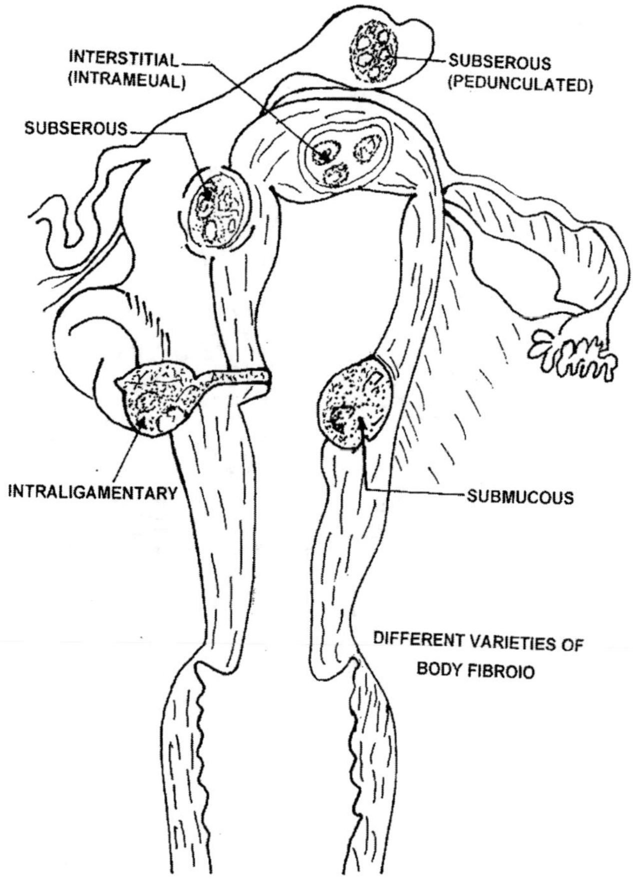

Fibroids

had abdominal discomfort which she thought was due to gastro intestinal upset. As the discomfort persisted ultrasound was done and to her surprise and her relatives it revealed an ovarian tumour with fluid in the abdomen. Cancer had already spread to the neighbouring organs. Pain in the beginning is rare and later is due to the spread of disease in other parts. Despite surgery, radiotherapy and chemotherapy she was not cured and died within a year and she had no symptom before she was diagnosed as cancer of the ovary.

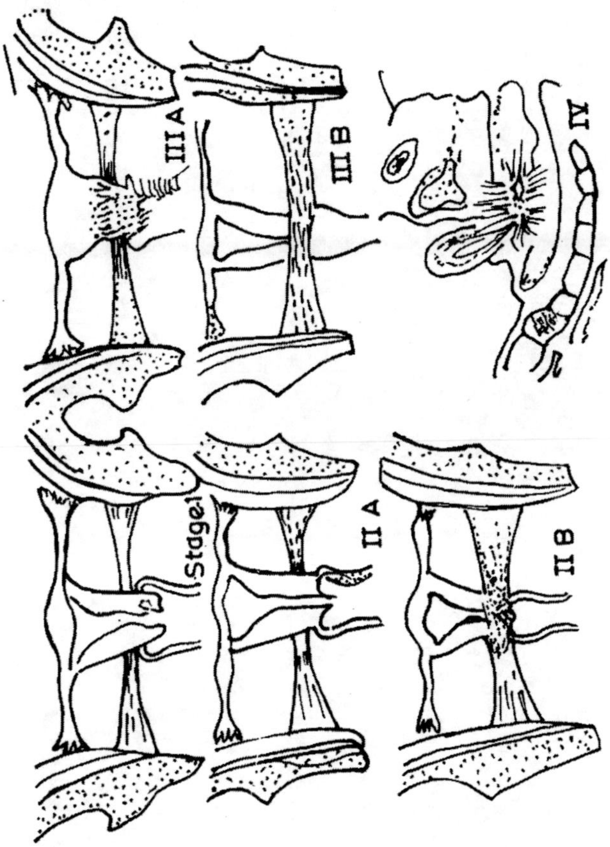

Stages of Carcinoma Cervix

45

ROLE OF RADIOTHERAPY IN THE TREATMENT OF CANCER

Dr. Radha Ghosh, M.S.

"Cancer", the very word sounds sinister. Until recently cancer was considered to be an incurable disease, and 'death' its ultimate fate. Medical science in the recent years has undergone great advancement. This has provided a better understanding of the disease process and of the tumor biology. Equipped with modern diagnostic aids, it is possible today to diagnose cancer at an early stage. Today, with better treatment facilities and advanced technology, some cancers can be cured at an early stage, while most cancers can be controlled, providing good palliation even at an advanced stage.

Cancer or a malignant growth is an abnormal proliferation of the cells of the body itself, which has escaped from the normal regulatory mechanism. The proliferation continues unabated, irrespective of the need of the organ. The growth continues to invade through normal tissues into distant organs. What causes this aberrated growth is till not very clear. Certain factors acting at the genetic and molecular level in association with some other causative factors like smoking, tobacco chewing, exposure to radiation, etc., may be responsible for transforming these benign cells into malignant ones.

The use of ionizing radiation in treating various disease entities mainly cancer is called Radiotherapy. As the word implies, ionizing radiation causes ionization of the water molecules of the cells. These free radicals produced as a result of ionization in turn initiates a series of chemical reactions which interferes with the vital functions of the cells. This may result in immediate death of the cell or may cause a permanent change in the genetic make-up of the cell, which may be transmitted in the next generation. Sometimes the damage is minimum and can be repaired fully. Which of these outcomes is effected depends on the dose delivered and the sensitivity of the cells. Low dose radiation mostly causes a change in the genetic type as it may be below the threshold for cell death. Most marked effects of radiation are on the cells of the gut and the bone marrow, as these cells have high mitotic index, that is, these cells divide rapidly. For the same reason, cancerous cells which are characterized by rapid proliferation, are also effected by radiation, while normal cells escape cell death. There exists a very narrow margin between the tumour lethal dose and tissue necrosis. Meticulous planning is therefore essential to provide adequate dose to the tumour, while preserving the vital functions of normal cells. Some amount of post-radiation complication is unavoidable.

The complications of radiation can be either immediate or delayed. In therapeutic doses the immediate complications encountered by patients are in the form of radiation sickness that is nausea, vomiting, vertigo, etc. The skin reactions usually seen during the course of treatment are in the form of redness dry desquamation or peeling of the skin progressing to wet desquamation. The late complications of radiation are fibrosis and lymphoedema. Severe radiation burns later on causing scarring and fibrosis are only seen with deep X-rays. Fortunately with megavoltage radiation, skin reactions specially the late reactions are not very common.

The tolerance of the small intestine is very low, and enteritis is a common complaint of patients receiving abdominal radiation. Sub-acute intestinal obstruction, acute intestinal obstruction, intestinal perforations are some of the late complications and are found mostly in patients with previous abdominal surgeries.

Patients receiving radiation in the head and neck areas experience mucositis which may be at times severe. Xerostomia or dryness of mouth is a late complication.

Radiation cystitis and proctitis are long-term complications encountered in patients treated by radiotherapy for cancer cervix.

The gonads, that is, the ovaries and the testis are the most vulnerable organs as far as radiation is concerned. Sometimes the ovaries are transpositioned into the abdominal cavity to preserve ovarian function. The male patients are advised to take the help of the sperm bank for need in future.

The use of computers in planning of radiotherapy has greatly helped to minimize the dose going to normal tissues, at the same time delivering adequate dose to the tumour, so as to effect a better control of the disease with minimum complications.

Cancer in general can be treated by three different modalities—Radiotherapy, Surgery and Chemotherapy. In early stages most cancers can be controlled by either radiation or surgery but as the disease progresses a multimodality approach has to be adopted for the better response and control.

Ionizing radiation has been in use for treating cancer for more than 100 years now. Radiotherapy is given in two forms:

(i) Teletherapy—meaning treatment from a distance.

(ii) Brachytherapy—meaning treatment from within a cavity in or around the tumour.

In the olden days, deep X-rays in the orthovoltage range were used for teletherapy purposes, but in the modern times are replaced by X-rays or photons of megavoltage range. These photons are produced in the Linear Accelerators, in the range of 4 MV to 25 MV. The main advantage of Megavoltage radiation over orthovoltage range are:

(i) the skin sparing effect

(ii) much improved depth doses

(iii) smaller extra dose to soft tissue elements of the bone, so less chances of osteoradionecrosis.

Linear Accelerators can also be designed for production of both photons and electrons.

Electrons owing to their special properties are used in treating superficial tumours, like that of the skin, the chest flap after mastectomy in breast cancer, boosting neck nodes, etc.

Whereas the Linear Accelerators produce X-rays or photons, 'Gamma-Ray Beam' units use a gamma-emitting radioactive nuclide to produce gamma rays. Owing to the decay of the radioactive source, it has to be replaced from time to time. Early Teletherapy units used Radium as the gamma-ray emitter, but the high photon energy made the protection of the source housing difficult. Besides the constant threat of a potential leakage of Radon gas made the use of Radium quite unsafe. For these reasons Radium has been largely replaced by Cobalt-60 and Ceasium-137.

Ceasium-137 has along half life but relatively low output dose rate. So it is rarely used in the Teletherapy units and has largely replaced Radium in the field of Brachytherapy.

Cobalt-60 is the most widely used isotope in the 'Gamma-Ray Beam' units. The effective photon energy of Cobalt-60 is only slightly lower than that of Radium. This advantage outweighs its short half-life. It is produced by nuclear bombardment of Cobalt-59.

Brachytherapy is given in the form of:

(i) Mould therapy

(ii) Iterstitial implants

(iii) Intracavitary treatment

Radioactive materials like Caesium-137, Cobalt-60, Iridium-192, Gold-198 are widely used in the form of tubes, needles seeds or pellets.

Iridium-192 has a very shor half-life of 74 days. It is used in the form of wires and pins for manual after loading and in the pellet form for remote after loading.

Gold-198 and Iodine-125 come in the form of grains and seeds and are used for permanent implants.

The manual insertion of preloaded sources into or around the tumour gives rise to high radiation exposure to the treating and attending personnel. To minimize such radiation hazards Remote After Loading Systems are rapidly replacing the older methods of manual preloading systems.

Fortunately most of the common types of cancers encountered in India are curable if diagnosed and treated at an early state.

Cancer of the Uterine Cervix is the most common cancer seen in women. It is treated by a combination of Teletherapy and Brachytherapy with a median 5 year survival of almost 80-90 per cent in the early stages.

Breast cancer is the next common cancer encountered in women. In early stages of the disease, removal of the lump followed by radiotherapy is all that is required. This helps in preserving the organ as well as maintaining the cosmoses and psychosis of the patient. In the advanced stages of course the effected breast has to be radiotherapy started along with has to control the disease effectively.

Cancers effecting the different organs of the head and neck areas are also common due to the abuse of beetle and tobacco. Combination of teletherapy and Brachytherapy is quite effective in controlling these diseases in early stages. Moreover radical surgeries which are often mutilating can be avoided providing a better quality of life to the patient. In advanced stages, a combination of chemotherapy, radiotherapy and surgery is required to control the disease.

With long-term survival in patients treated with radiotherapy, delayed complications of radiation are encountered more frequently. It is therefore mandatory for patients to undergo regular check ups at any cancer clinic for prompt management of these complications.

In recent years, Intraoperative Radiotherapy and Radiosurgery are also very much in use and have shown some very promising and interesting results. In the coming years there are promising prospects for cancer patients.

46

BREAST CANCER

Dr. Vatsala Samant

Cancer is not a single disease, with a single cause and single type of treatment.

There are more than 200 types of cancers each with its own name and treatment. The causes of breast cancer are not completely understood but certain women do seem to be slightly at higher risk of developing the disease. Women with a family history of breast cancer particularly in their mother or sister, women who either have no children or have them late in life, women whose periods started when they were very young or when menopause occurred late, all seem to run a slightly greater risk. Women who took the earlier type of contraceptive pills may have a slightly greater chance of developing breast cancer than women who have never taken the pill.

Symptoms

Breast

(i) Change of size or shape

(ii) Dimpling of the skin

(iii) Lump or thicking

Nipples

(i) Discharge

(ii) Rash

(iii) Inversion or turning in

(iv) Lump or thicking

Arm swelling of armpit and arm

No Pain

In 90 per cent a lump on the breast is present.

Investigations

1. Mammography may be done.

2. Palpation of the breast which can be done during bathing. Quite a large number of lumps are detected by women themselves.

3. Doctors do needle aspiration of the lump as well as needle biopsy.

Treatment

(i) Surgery, radiotherapy, chemotherapy, and hormone therapy.

(ii) Surgery—lumpectomy or removal of the lump.

(iii) Mastactomy—either simple or radical lymph glands removal.

(iv) Radiotherapy—irradiation either externally or internally.

(v) Hormone Therapy—Hormones are substances that occur naturally in the body, and control the growth and activity of normal cells.

The female hormones oestrogen and progesterone can affect the growth of breast cancer cells. Hormone therapy for breast cancer consists in effect of anti-hormonal treatment to prevent female hormones working on the breast cancer cells.

Chemotherapy

Use of anti-cancer drugs to destroy cancer cells and so these drugs interrupt the growth and division of cells. Chemotherapy is generally started after surgery either orally or intravenously.

Ill-Effects: The drug affects not only cancer cells but also the normal cells of the body and thus the immune system and one becomes vulnerable to infection. There can be nausea, vomiting, diarrhea, hair loss, stomatitis and ulcer in the mouth. After some time these symptoms disappear. Men can also have cancer of the breast but it is rare.

Advice

If you notice a lump in your breast do not delay visiting your doctor. Also anything unusual seen or felt in your breast must be examined because even though most breast lumps are benign they still need to be checked to rule out the possibility of cancer. Because if the lump is cancer the earlier the treatment starts the better the chances of cure. I have known cases of breast cancer completely cured.

Transplant Therapy for Breast Cancer

A new controversial breast cancer therapy which is the most potent weapon is, high doses of chemotherapy accompanied by a transplant of stem cells which are precursors of disease immune fighting stem cells. The transplant therapy is preliminary, though people claim that with treatment at least some people have survived.

The technique is to flood the body with toxic chemotherapy drugs in an effort to overwhelm the malignancy. Though the drug does kill the cancer cells it also destroys most of the disease fighting cells of the immune system. Marrow cells from the bones or stem cells from the blood steam are harvested, both of which give rise to new cells before they begin chemotherapy. When the treatment is done these cells are reinfused into body in the hope that the immune systems will rebound.

Self-Examination

You should examine your breasts regularly, to check for possible signs of cancer, you must do this every month immediately after periods or, if you have had the menopause, on the first day of each month. There may be difference in the size or shape of the breasts. Prominent veins may be there on the breasts.

Detect Breast Cancer Early

Breast cancer is the second most common cancer in Indian women. If detected early, it can be readily treated. Unfortunately many patients report to their doctors six months after the first signs appear. Most breast diseases are not cancerous. But only a proper and systematic examination can help the patient to know whether it is cancer or not. Therefore as a first step learn to examine yourself regularly for signs of breast disease. Early detection and early treatment will save many lives.

When to Suspect Breast Disease

- Swelling, thickening, or lumps in any part of the breast
- Discharge or bleeding from the nipple
- Change in shape of nipple

- Any ulcer which does not heal
- Dimpling of skin over the breast
- Lumps in the armpit

There are several factors which are associated with an increased risk (high risk category) for developing breast cancer. They are:

1. Women whose mothers or sisters have had breast cancer.
2. Those who have had cancer in one breast, the other breast is at risk.
3. Women who have never had children, or who have had their first child after 30 years age.
4. Women who have fibrocystic disease of the breast.

How to Detect Cancer Early

- Every woman above 35 years of age should examine her breasts herself every month, on the day her period ends.
- Ideally every woman above 50 years of age should have an annual examination by a doctor. Mammography may be done routinely once a year, or when adviced.
- If you are in the high-risk category for breast cancer, mammography can detect very early breast cancer even before symptoms appear, and thus gives a better chance for cure. For high risk women, annual mammographic screening is recommended after 40 years of age.

What is Mammography?

It is an X-ray of the breast done with a special X-ray machine. The breast has to be compressed (flattened out) a little and then the X-ray is taken. It is not a painful procedure, although some women experience some discomfort due to the compression, especially if done just before their periods. Hence it is recommended that mammography be done after the periods are over. Mammography is useful in detecting early breast lumps before they can be felt by the patient or doctor, as well as to determine the nature of any lump that is felt. Mammography should be done on the advice of a treating doctor.

47

DEFENCE SYSTEMS OF THE BODY

Dr. Vatsala Samant

Our body is a superb example of the working of various systems in a coordinated fashion so as to make us live an enjoyable life. It is the grandest and the most complex machine ever built. Unfortunately we take it far too much for granted, unless something goes wrong. Knowledge of our body, its organs and systems and how they work to maintain our health and fitness is essential.

We are made up from a tiny cell or fertilized egg which goes on dividing cells and an embryo is formed with its various organs and systems. Cell is the basic element of life and we have about 60 trillions of cells organized into power station, transportation system and a sophisticated communication set-up. Raw materials are manufactured into useful goods and a garbage disposal system, an efficient government, a rigid dictatorship and a defence system keep out and fight undesirable invaders. The cell story can be summed up thus: these 60 trillion cells can live in harmony, each minding its own business and each performing its own task. This is a supreme wonder. No doubt our defence system cannot be visualized. It consists of natural barriers and a complicated immune system.

We live surrounded by plant and animal kingdoms, bacteria, viruses, chemical poisons, and we have to fight these if we want to enjoy life. First let us deal with the natural basics:

The skin which covers our body is a rampart, protecting against mighty hordes of potentially deadly invading bacteria. The skin's outer layer prevents the entry of the germs. Sweat secreted by the skin glands is acidic and further prevents the establishment of bacteria. The skin also has friendly bacteria flourishing. Waste products of these bacteria inhibit growth of invading germs.

Similarly, our sweat, tears and saliva have an enzyme that kills the germs. So also the gastric juice of the stomach. Also the line hair in the nostrils filter the air from the bacteria and those that escape the nose are filtered by the mucous lining of the respiratory system.

The second and the most important line of defence is our immune system. It fights against bacteria, viruses, fungi, harmful germs cells, poisons and foreign transplants which have come as a relief to the organs like kidney, liver, etc. Our immune and defence systems are more complete than the defence system of any country. There are two kinds of immune systems and both can be distinguished between self and non-self. They are:

1. Humoural
2. Cell medicated

Our blood contains two kinds of cells—red and white. Red blood cells carry oxygen. It is the white blood cells which are our weapons against the invaders. They beat bacteria and virus. White blood cells are about 7000 per mm and are of various forms like polymorphs, lymphocytes, etc. Of these lymphocytes are the most important to fight the enemy.

The scenario is that of the battlefield with the bacteria and the virus fighting the white blood cells. Invading germs have foreign molecules which form antigen poison for our body cell. The white blood cells get into action immediately and produce antibodies and neutralize the antigens.

Lymphocytes are major cells of defence and are of two types—B and T. The B cells are formed in the bone marrow and through the thymus—a tiny gland behind the sternum. B cell converts into plasma cells. Plasma cells liberate antibodies which circulate in the tissue fluids. Antibodies adhere to the surface of the bacteria and speed up their destruction and neutralize toxins produced by bacterias. This process is known as humeral immune response. Further polymorphs of the blood cells complete the destruction.

T Lymphocytes are the main weapons to fight the invaders. There are three types of T cells:

1. Killer
2. Helper
3. Suppresser.

Killer T cells destroy infected cells, viruses, cancer cells and tissue cells of the transplant. But there is a virus—HIV—which kills or attacks the T cells and destroys them and these cells are thrown into circulation and infect the body cells and the entire immune system becomes inefficient and the body succumbs to various diseases. This is what is known as AIDS.

Helper T cell helps B Lymphocytes in their action of destruction of the invaders and regulates the body's defence mechanism.

Suppresser T cell suppresses the total immune system and is instrumental in preventing antibody being produced against the invaders.

This whole phenomenon is known as cell medicated defence system.

48

AIDS

Dr. Vatsala Samant

Acquired (not congenital) immunity (body defence system) deficiency (no weapon to fight the virus) syndrome virus known as HIV is responsible to cause this disease. AIDS was first recognized in USA in 1981 though it was quite rampant in Africa. Only the human beings are affected and some apes but it is absent in any other mammalians. It is a sexually transmitted disease. First it was noticed in homosexual people but as early as 1990, cases of AIDS were seen in people other than homosexuals such as male, female injecting drug users, recipients of the donor of HIV contaminated blood, heterosexual men and women, including sex workers and infants born to infected women.

Unfortunately there are no initial symptoms or signs of the disease but in time to come any illness affecting the infected person is prolonged because the body immune system is paralysed by the virus and ultimately being unable to recover the person dies. In the early stages symptoms are vague—weight loss, fever, diarrhoea. Later the person is affected by pneumonia and skin cancer. AIDS has a duration of five years of incubation period. The average life span of the AIDS victim is less than eight months from the date of hospitalization. Studies show that women are getting affected more rapidly and at an earlier age than men. Further studies show that:

1. Women are increasingly becoming infected with HIV. In most of the Third World, the number of infected women is as many as or more than the infected men.

2. Women are becoming infected at a significantly younger age than men. On an average, they become infected five to ten years earlier than men.

3. Proportionately more girls and young women in their teens and twenties are becoming infected than women in any other age group. Even post-menopause women are susceptible to HIV infections. The implications are that it is possible that women become more infected than men. For most women the major risk for HIV infection is due to young age of marriage, first pregnancy or sexual intercourse. The growing number of women infected or dying is of great concern and must sound an alarm. Women are also at increased risk of being infected by HIV through contaminated blood transfusions associated with pregnancy, anaemia, post partum haemorrhage, ectopic pregnancy and abortions.

HIV infection is preventable but dependency on husband and thus powerlessness strips a woman to protect herself. It is always the husband who is the vector for HIV infection for which HIV preventive measures such as the condom that inhibit conception are not acceptable.

Preventive measures are: reduction in the number of sexual partners, monogamy, safer sexual practice, use of condoms.

Diagnosis and treatment is possible only when women and men can present themselves to someone with the skills and measures to identify correctly their conditions and supply appropriate medicines. Laboratory HIV was isolated in 1984 and tests for HIV became common and available in 1985. Compared to any other disease, the issues related to the diagnosis of HIV are more complex. AIDS is invariably fatal and infection is lifelong. Dr Jonas Salk who developed an effective vaccine against polio has developed a vaccine against HIV. Though AIDS is a tougher target than polio Dr Salk's new treatment is given to people already infected with HIV as one shot every three months. According to some doctors however there is no evidence that the vaccine does any good. Dr Peachers used blood from the placenta in the treatment of Leukaemia in children because the immune cells in a newborn have not learnt to attack foreign proteins. This treatment was successful in young patients. They believe this technique can be applied to other diseases like AIDS in ten years, as the technique could also oust the damaged immune system of AIDS patients provided the scientists first find out a way to disrupt the reproductive cycle of AIDS, if the virus can be controlled, the immune system can be replaced.

In 1989 AZT was okayed as treatment for AIDS. There is another drug protase combined with AZT which has a better effect on HIV. In America today, many teenagers are staying in the shadow of AIDS, the terrifying modern epidemic that travels by blood in the bodies' immune system. A virus that causes invariably a fatal disease, but today the AZT and Protase injection has helped to lift death sentence for a few years at least and perhaps longer, on millions of AIDS sufferer's. AIDS itself can be the trigger for cancer directly causing cells to turn malignant.

49

SEX EDUCATION

Dr. Vatsala Samant

One of the most widely discussed subjects today in schools and colleges, by State Governments and social organisations, and among parents, is whether to introduce sex education into the teaching institutions or not. Our bodies work methodically, and have various systems: nervous, digestive, excretory, etc., and only one system the reproductive which is completely ignored and misunderstood. We are living today as a result of the reproductive system and yet we neglect it.

Our other systems start working with the beginning of life. Our circulatory system for instance. The heart starts working even when the baby in the womb. The digestive system starts at birth, and though it can only digest mother's milk at first, gradually it develops to digest solid food. But the reproductive system is quite quiescent until puberty. There are changes in the body and the mind, and it is better that young people be told about the facts of life, because they are stepping into that stage of life when they become capable of reproducing their kind. Because of this they face new risks to their health and well-being.

Girls and boys after a certain age come to know about sex, either through friends, school mates or by reading in books. The question is whether what they learn is correct or not.

The spread of AIDS has brought this subject of sex education to the forefront. Other sexually transmitted diseases STD are also a threat. Normally our body is capable of fighting a disease through its immune system, with the help of the white blood cells, etc. In AIDS this immune system becomes deficient. A person suffering from the HI Virus which causes this disease, loses the capacity to fight any disease faces suffering and dies.

Education is the only tool available to inform our school children with correct knowledge of the scientific aspects of reproduction. It is the only way to alert them to the danger of these disease.

There are many cases of ignorance and misconceptions among girls and boys which cause needless trauma. Yet parents oppose sex education in the school curriculum, even if they are not able to convey this information to their children themselves. In the 1994, third Asian Sexology Conference, a survey was done among the Delhi colleges, and only one-third of the students could correctly answer questions on sex. About 47 per cent said they had learnt sex from friends and only 5 per cent said they learnt from their parents.

The onset of menstruation in a girl who is uninformed, arouses emotions of fear and shame, and can give her a psychological shock from which she may never fully recover. Boys should also have a full knowledge of sex. Parents think that sex education will corrupt young minds. Failure of adolescents to realize the implications and potential dangers of sex can lead to tragedy. Sex education should come naturally. Children invariably ask questions and these should be answered simply but truthfully. Sex education should be a part of the general knowledge of the child, acquired in the course of family conversation.

There should be no harm if it is taught factually in school? The WHO published a report in 1992 that revealed that more than two-thirds of the population between the ages of 14 to 19 in developing countries have had at least one sexual experience, and this is the age group most vulnerable to suffer from STDs. Reports claim that 20 to 25 per cent of HIV infections are likely to occur in the age group of those under 25. Parents, instead of opposing sex education in school should insist on it, to arm their children and protect them against deadly disease like AIDS.

Madhya Pradesh and some Municipal schools in Bombay had introduced sex education but as is the practice in our political set up, the opposition raised objections to it.

Under the modern conditions, there comes a time when all girls and boys may benefit from formal instruction in the physiology of reproduction, and of the pitfalls which accompany the unbridled urge. Such teaching could come naturally into the school curriculum, as a part of a course on health education. Knowledge of the facts often leads to postponing the initiation of intercourse and sexual activity.

Let us not hide the facts of life from our children who in due course of time will be the architects of future generations.

There are reports that early sex education imparted in schools has its adverse affects also. Adolescents after being aware of sex have started experiencing it, which, is a very negative aspect of sex education. All aspects should be very carefully studied before imparting it at a younger age.

50

HORMONES

Dr. Vatsala Samant

Our body has a variety of glands. Mainly there are two types of glands. Glands with ducts and glands without ducts. Examples of the first variety are the breast and salivary glands. All these pour their secretions through a duct. The other variety is of ductless ones which have their secretions directly mingled in the blood circulation and these secretions are known as Hormones. There are large number of ductless glands producing hormones but the most important are the Pituitary, Ovaries and Thyroid. These cause development of reproductive track, orchestrate menses, pregnancy, menopause, maintain general health of women as well as physiological events in a woman's life.

Pituitary

It is situated at the base of the brain and is divided into two parts—posterior and anterior. Anterior part is responsed in the production of a number of hormones that have a profound effect both positively and negatively on the control of growth of a child development of secondary sexual characters, and this hormone is known as growth hormone. Even pituitary is under control of hypothalamus, a part of the brain. Growth hormone and growth failure represents one of the remedial cause of severe short stature. Primary dwarfism is due to congenital hypoplasia of anterior pituitary gland in which there is short stature, genital hypoplasia, absence of pubic hair, and ammenorrhoea. Functional anterior pituitary disorders, obesity is a constant feature, in the infantile form sex retardation is well marked. Sex organs remain immature after the age of puberty and secondary sex characters are absent. Pituitary gland also produces stimulating hormones of the ovary and thyroid gland. Posterior part produces pitocin which causes contraction of the uterus and is always used in the third stage of childbirth to control post-partum bleeding. There can be benign or malignant tumours of the pituitary gland which can be diagnosed by CAT scan.

Ovarion Hormones

Ovary, the sex gland besides producing and storing millions of eggs, produces hormones—oestrogen and progestrone. These hormones are responsible for growth of the reproductive track, secondary sexual characters, orchestrating menstrual cycle and maintaining pregnancy. Deficiency of these hormones causes cardiac-osteodiseases. Oestrogen has a protective effect on these. Oestrogen gets reduced in amount at menopause. The other hormone progestrone is formed after ovulation and it forms corpus lueteum which is necessary to continue pregnancy. Both the hormones are under the control of anterior pituitary gland.

51

THYROID

Dr. Manjula Pande, M.S.

Thyroid gland is situated in the front of the neck. Normally in some cases there is a slight enlargement of the gland premenstrually without any symptoms. When thyroid is not working properly the condition is known as hypothyroidism and thyroid hormone is less and on the other hand when it is overworking the condition is known as hyperthyroidism and when there is enlargement of the gland the condition is known as goitre.

Hypothyroidism. There is retention of fluid causing swelling all over the body, a condition known as myxeoedima. There are menstrual disorders, intolerance of heat, fatigue, etc. It is common at places where there is lack of iodine in the water.

Treatment is to give Thyroxane

Hyperthyroidism. It is the condition resulting from the effect of excessive amount of circulating thyroid hormone on the body tissue.

Symptoms

Nervousness, inability to get along with others, tremors, tachycardia, fast pulse, heart enlargement, heart failure in the later stage, weakness of the muscles, weight loss, impairment of fertility, feeling cold all the time, eyes show lid lag retract. Treatment is Antithyroid drug and thyroidectomy which is partial removal of the gland.

The thyroid is a small gland which has two tubes situated in the front of neck, weighing about 20-25 grams.

This gland secrets a hormone called Thyroxin which is responsible for maintaining the basic metabolism of the body.

An important substance required for the synthesis of Thyroxine is Iodine and lack of which will lead to deficiency of Thyroxine.

The thyroid hormone influences the growth and hypothyrodic maintenance of all body tissues, turn over of all substrates, vitamins, hormones and total energy expenditure in the body.

Diseases of the thyroid gland may be due to either of deficiency or over secretion of it's hormone.

The deficiency of thyroid hormone what is known as hypothyroidism can occure at any stage of life. If it occurs in childhood it can cause failure of physical and mental growth, delayed milestones, weight gain and lethargy. I have got a small girl aged six years who started menstruating on invcoting atives she was found to be a hypothyrodic child, treated accordingly and now she has stopped menstruation with improvement in her physical and mental state.

Hypothyridism at puberty can lead to short statue, retardation in sexual metneation, excessive weight gain and poor performance character menstruating at school may call attention to the diagnosis.

In the adult hypothyroidism may lead to lethargy, constipation, cold intolerance, muscle cramps, menstrual irregularity, weight gain, decline in appetite, loss of hair, horse voice, thick and coarse skin.

Hyperthyroidism on the other hand in when thyroid hormone is produced in excess and causes insomnia, nervousness, tremors, frequent loose stools, palpitation, decreased menstrual flow, weight loss despite of good appetite, can cause angina and the person appears anxious, restless, fidgety with wide bulging eyes.

There is mare more disease of thyroid where its functioning is normal but due to deficiency of iodine in the diet the thyroid enlarges and forms a swelling in front of the neck called goitre.

When detected in time thyroid abnormalities are treatable but may need prolonged or life long use of medicines.

At present working as consultant and Head of the Department of Obstetriest Gynaecology, Nazareth Hospital Allahabad.

Thyroid disorders are often common during pregnancy and post-barlium period and treatment is gratifying for mother and baby. Lack of thyroid hormone results in permanent physical and Mental retardation screening proytemme his starter in western countries to detect hypothyroid which is done a first few days of life. Hypothyroidism in adults is usually idoopathic cause not known early symptoms are viable, missed and classical symptoms may with month or years to appear.

Iodine deficiency is among the most widespread of all malnutritional disease and it causes permanent brain damage and mental retardation in children (reproductive failure decrease child survival, goitre and socio-economic stagnation.

52

FITNESS

Dr. Vatsala Samant

Fitness means clean skin, bright eyes, slim body, correct weight according to your height, walking straight, lifting weight, breathing properly, thinking rationally, without much of stress, etc.

The most important factor needed to life take a happy life is one's fitness or to be fit. Fitness is not necessary just to be happy, but also to achieve success in life and physical, mental, moral, spiritual attainment. It is one's duty to be fit for oneself, one's family and one's country.

First we must think of how to keep fit so that illness can be avoided because if you are fit and healthy, diseases will have no opportunity to attack you and if attacked, your defence system being fit and you can defeat the disease.

To remain fit one must know about diet. A healthy person to remain fit does not eat unless hungry and eats only what is required by the body, i.e., caloric estimation about 3000 calories if working and 2500 if sedentary. To remain fit one has to live in pure environment, sleep soundly and get up in the morning feeling fresh and full of energy to be ready for the day's work. After the days work, the fatigue that one feels is responsible for deep sleep..

Thus, to live a healthy and fit life from its beginning till end should be the aim of all people.

Necessary Elements of Diet

Fibre

Fibre are of two kinds—one is from cereals which are slightly inferior and second variety is from fruits and vegetables which are supposed to produce reduction in cholesterol and so are beneficial for cases of heart disease.

Fat

There are two types of fats. Saturated found in animal products and dairy products and the other variety unsaturated found in vegetables and these are suppose to lesson the risk of heart disease. Hormones necessary for growth and reproduction are produced by cholesterol and cholesterol is produced by our body cells. Excess cholesterol remains in the blood steam and clings to the walls of our arteries as fatty deposits and that obstructs the blood flow and later on, leads to heart disease. So to avoid heart disease one should eat less fatty food.

Fat should constitute 3 per cent of a healthy diet. They are highly concentrated energy source and are necessary or vital to the process of cell growth and repair of our body cells.

Proteins

Amino acids are building blocks in the formation of new cells and are provided by protein intake in our diet. Proteins are needed in greater amounts during pregnancy and lactation all enzymes are also protein. Deficiency of protein result in the retardation of body growth, loss of culaneous and fat leading to dry skin. Deficiency leads to mental changes. Liver gets enlarged and there is anaemia. But very high protein diet strains the kidneys. Protein help in the body growth and repair, replacement of body tissues, muscles and bones. Protein are found in cereals dals, cereals and meat, fish and eggs are very rich in protein.

Carbohydrates

Rice, sugar, potatoes, bread, flour, are rich in carbohydrate which give us energy.

Starch is present in cereals, pulses, nuts, seeds, and roots, sweet potatoes and beet root. They are required for the oxidation of fats and also in bringing about nervous activity.

Minerals

We need salts of various types, some are required in large quantity and others in traces. There are about 20 different minerals that play a role in combating bodies metabolism.

Macronutrients

Chief are Potassium, Sodium, Phosphorus, Calcium and Magnesium.

Micronutrients

Iron, Copper, Zinc, Iodine.

Minerals are highly essential. Calcium is present in bone and teeth. Iron is present in haemoglobin and lack of it causes anaemia.

Potasium: present in orange, controls water balance.

Sodium: in common salt.

Iodine: helps in formation of Thyroid hormone.

ESSENTIAL MINERALS

Mineral	*Essential for*	*Source*
Sodium	Formation of body tissues including blood	Table salt, vegetable
Calcium	Formation of bones and teeth. Needed for proper functioning of heart, nerves and for clotting of blood	Milk, cereals, vegetables, grams, meat
Phosphorus	Formation of bones and ATP also for DNA duplication	Milk, cereals, grain, vegetables
Magnesium	Action of muscles and nerves	Vegetables
Potasium	For body growth and blood function	Vegetables
Iron	Haemoglobin	Meat, liver, green vegetables
Iodine	Production of thyroid secretion	Sea food, water salts

Water

60 per cent of our body weight is water and major constitution of it performs several functions. It helps in the absorption of cells substances, maintain body balance.

Vitamins

A balanced diet must contain all the vitamins we need and are essential for the proper growth.

A_1 is necessary for formation of bones, teeth and to keep skin and hair healthy and is also essential for the eyes.

B_1 promotes production of energy and is needed for proper functioning of the nerves, muscles and heart.

B_2 helps to stimulate the release of energy for nutrients, keep, skin, mouth, tongue healthy, helps in hormone produce.

Vitamin B_6 helps in the formation of red blood cells and antibodies and also helps digestive system.

B_{12} essential for formation of new cells.

Vitamin C maintains teeth, bones, blood vessels and helps the immune system of the body.

Vitamin D aids in calcium absorption from food and is responsible for strong teeth and bones.

Vitamin E assists in the formation of red blood cells and slows down ageing of cells.

Acupuncture

Acupuncture is an ancient chinese healing art it aims to restore the smooth flow of Qi means a sense of fullness distention & mild electric shock. Though this energy circulates within the body it can be accessed at many superficial points located along the major meridians. Each of these meridians is associated with specific organs & every acupuncture point is considered to have a particular therepeutic effect.

There are 365 acupuncture points but according to some the total of acupuncture points are more than 2000. Acupuncturists select points on patients body & insert needles & also some of them use other theraputic techniques not all if which recquire the insertion of needless.

The method consists of insertion of one slender needle at each selected point & the needles are turirebod for greater stimulation, some use weak electric current sent throught the conventional needles to produce the sam effect. this method is useful when continued stimulate (15 to 20 minutes) of a point is indicated.

Acupuncture points can also be stimulated by heat pressure. Some times small cones if herban placed in these needless & are buned to produce penetrating heat & are removed before causing pain.

Deep finger pressure known as acupuncture is used by some acupuncturists. it can be used to relieve headache & menstrual discomfort or dysmanorrbean.

Acupuncture is supposed to relieve pain seen be used preventively & therapeticaly. There is a belonging treatments to avert cold & flu with climatic changes.

The never use of acupuncture is acupuncute analyesia which is used surgery.

By far the most common use for acupuncture is in the treatment of chronic pain people have reported relief from intractable conditions as arthirities, chronic headaches & back pain. It has also been used for treatment of drug addiction, Alcoholism & even smoking. How does acupuncture works. Some physicologist suggest that it works by stimulating the body's production if various pain blocking neurd chemicals the effectiveness of the treatment seems to depend on which pomts are stimulated. Nedeling at the stage of pain prompts the spinal cord to generate chemicals that work locally.

Diet During Pregnancy

Physical and mental health of the mother during pregnancy has an influence on the growth of the foetus and so nutrition during pregnancy is very important. Former view that the mother needs to "eat for two" or double quantity is out of date. The five basic food elements, proteins, fats, carbohydrates, minerals and vitamins are all necessary to maintain mother's health during pregnancy. Iron is deficient in our diet particularly those from the poor class where anaemia is almost endemic and so during pregnancy some iron in some form has to be taken by the pregnant woman and so also calcium. If milk is taken in any form during pregnancy: supplies the necessary calcium needed for the body.

Wheat *roti,* rice, *dal,* vegetable, salads, fruits guava or banana and six glasses of water is a must for the woman. Meat, fish, eggs can be taken but not everyday.

It is very difficult to prescribe a balanced diet. It depends on various factors such as age, sex, physiological condition and nature of profession of individual. The energy requirements differs with age and profession. Old sedintary people need 2500 calories to teenagers and people working hard 3500 calories.

VITAMIN AND THEIR ROLE

Vitamin, daily requirement	***Sources***	***Needed for***	***Deficiency disorders***
A_1 (Retinol) 1 mg	Fish, liver, egg butter, vegetable cheese	Skin, eyes, bones internal organs	Retardation of growth, night blindness, Xeropthalmia
B_1 (Thiamine) 1.5 mg	Milk, cheese, whole cereals	Carbohydrates, metabolism and	Retardation of growth, Beri beri

	vegetables, fruits yeast, milk	energy release	
B_2 (Riboflavin) 1.5 mg	Milk, cheese, green vegetables, fruits, liver, fish	Tissue repair and healthy skin	Retardation of growth, inflammation of tongue, scaly skin
B_6 (Pyridoxin) 2 mg	Whole grains, liver yeast, vegetables	Healthy teeth, gums blood vessels, Rbcs	Skin diseases in chick and rat
Folic acid 0.4 mg	Green leafy vegetables yeast meat, fish	RBC production	Anaemia
Biotin 0.2 mg	Egg yolk, nuts, liver, kidney, fresh vegetables	Healthy circulatory system and skin	Deficiency usually does not occur in humans
C (Ascorbic acid) 50 mg	Fruits (esp. lemon, orange) vegetables	Tissue metabolism wound healing	Scurvy, defective teeth, loss of calcium
D_2 (ergocalci-ferol) 0.01 mg	Fish, butter, sunlight	Calcium and phosphorus metabolism	Rickets, defective teeth, bone disease
E (Tocophenol) 10 mg	Green vegetables wheat, milk, butter, whole cereals	Maintaining cell membrane	Sterility in rats No deficiency in humans
K (0.1 mg)	Green vegetables	Clotting of blood	Deficiency does not occur in humans

An adult should have at least 1000 mg calcium everyday.

FOODS RICH IN CALCIUM

Food	*Quantity*	*Calorie mg*
Cows milk	240 gm	288
Yoghurt (dahi)	200gm	298
Kulfei (Buffaloo milk)	100 gm	525
Dry coconut	100gm	400
Dry dates	100gm	120
Black currants	100gm	130

Other Calcium Foods

Cottage cheese, jaggery, soyabean, cauliflower, dried shrimps and Sardines.

All the values are per 100 g. of edible portion.

Name of the Foodstuff	*Protein (g.)*	*Fat (g.)*	*Carbohydrates (g.)*
Cereal Grains:			
Bajra	11.6	5.0	67.5
Jowar	10.4	1.9	72.6
Ragi	7.3	1.3	72.0

Rice	6.8	0.5	78.2
Rice flakes	6.6	1.2	77.3
Rice puffed	7.5	0.1	73.6
Wheat Hour	12.1	1.7	69.4
Semolina (Rava)	10.4	0.8	74.8
Vermicelli	8.7	0.4	78.3
Brown Bread	8.8	1.4	49.0
White Bread	7.8	0.7	51.9
Pulses and Legumes:			
Chana dal	20.8	5.3	60.9
Uelid dal	24.0	1.4	59.6
Mung dal	24.5	1.2	59.9
Whole mung	24.0	1.3	56.7
Tur dal	22.3	1.7	57.6
Lentil (Masoor)	25.1	0.7	59.0
Peas (dry)	19.7	1.1	56.5
Rajmah	22.9	1.3	60.6
Leafy Veg.:			
Corriander	3.3	0.6	6.3
Fenugreek	4.4	0.9	6.0
Lettuce	2.1	0.3	2.5
Mint	4.8	0.6	5.8
Spinach	2.0	0.7	2.9
Radish Leaves	3.8	0.4	2.4
Roots and Tubers:			
Beetroot	1.7	0.1	8.8
Carrot	0.9	0.2	10.6
Onion (big)	1.2	0.1	11.1
Potato	1.6	0.1	22.6
Sweet Potato	1.2	0.3	28.2
Yam	1.4	0.1	26.0
Other Veg.:			
Bottle gourd	0.2	0.1	2.5
Brinjal	1.4	0.3	4.0
Broad Beans	4.5	0.1	7.2
Cauliflower	2.6	0.4	4.0
Cluster Beans	3.2	0.4	10.8
Cucumber	0.4	0.1	2.5

Capsicum	1.3	0.3	4.3
Ladies fingers	1.9	0.2	6.4
Pumpkin	1.4	0.1	4.6
Parwar	2.0	0.3	2.2
Snake gourd	0.5	0.3	3.3
Tinde	1.4	0.2	3.4
Nuts and Oilseeds:			
Almond	20.8	58.9	10.5
Cashewnut	21.2	46.9	22.3
Coconut (dry)	6.8	62.3	18.4
Coconut (fresh)	4.5	41.6	13.0
Coconut water	1.4	0.1	4.4
Til	18.3	43.3	25.0
Groundnut	25.3	40.1	26.1
Walnut	15.6	64.5	11.0
Fruits :			
Amla	0.5	0.1	13.7
Apple	0.2	0.5	13.4
Banana (ripe)	1.2	0.3	27.2
Cherries (red)	1.1	0.5	13.8
Dates (dried)	2.5	0.4	75.8
Dates (fresh)	1.2	0.4	33.8
Figs	1.3	0.2	7.6
Grapes	0.5	0.3	16.5
Guava	0.9	0.3	11.2
Sweet lime	0.8	0.3	9.3
Water melon	0.2	0.2	3.3
Fruits:			
Lichi	1.1	0.2	13.6
Mango (ripe)	0.6	0.4	16.9
Musk melon	0.3	0.2	3.5
Orange	0.7	0.2	10.9
Papaya	0.6	0.1	7.2
Peaches	1.2	0.3	10.5
Pine Apple	0.4	0.1	10.8
Sapota	0.7	1.1	21.4
Sitaphal	1.6	0.4	23.5
Tomato (ripe)	0.9	0.2	3.6

Fish and other sea food:			
Pomfrets (black)	20.3	2.6	1.5
Pomfrets (white)	17.0	1.3	1.8
Prawn	19.1	1.0	0.8
Ravas	22.2	1.1	3.3
Sardine	21.0	1.9	-
Surmai	19.9	1.4	-
Meat and Poultry:			
Egg (hen)	13.3	13.3	-
Food	25.9	0.6	-
Mutton	18.5	13.3	-
Beef (muscle)	79.2	10.3	0.2
Pork (muscle)	18.7	4.4	-
Milk and Milk Products:			
Milk (cow's)	3.2	4.1	4.4
Milk (Buffalo's)	4.3	6.5	5.0
Skim milk pd.	38.0	0.1	51.0
Cheese	24.1	25.1	6.3
Fats and Oil:			
Butter	-	81.0	-
Cooking oil /ghee	-	100.0	-
Sugars:			
Honey	0.3	0	79.5
Jaggery (cane)	6.4	0.1	95.0
Miscellaneous:			
Sago	0.2	0.2	87.1
Neera	0.4	-	10.9
Sugarcane Juice	0.1	0.2	9.1

53

AEROBICS

Dr. Vatsala Samant

Aerobics are energetic type of exercises. Performed to music with a clear simple beat.

Advantage: Aerobics improves the efficiency of your heart, lungs, and as a result can help to reduce the risk of heart disease and circulation.

Action Plan: Aerobic exercise can be either high or low impact (the force with which the feet hit the ground). Start with low impact when one foot always stays on the ground and progress gradually to high impact if you wish.

Tips and Risks: People who have heart disease, overweight and who have problems with their lower back knees and ankles or hip should avoid any kind of impact particularly high impact.

54

EXERCISE AND DIET

Dr. Vatsala Samant

Fitness is a very important part of all human beings and their body. The more active you are the less likely you are to suffer from any diseases. Even a little exercise everyday is better than not doing any at all. Fitness slips away quite quickly. Once we stop regular exercise, our fitness starts declining. Exercise has to be for life. A survey was done in England and its report said "Activity and fitness matters revealed 80 per cent of the people believed they are fit and most of them were kidding themselves".

Advantages of Exercise

Exercise reduces chances of heart disease, strokes, improves circulation, makes muscles strong and joints flexible, keeps body weight down. People who exercise regularly develop self-confidence. By doing exercise regularly one gets sound sleep. When one gets ill then the recovery is also fast. Exercise may be vigorous or moderate like: swimming, running, tennis, dancing, etc.

Hints Before you Start

Don't try too much too soon. Don't under do it either. Don't exercise if you are ill. The right exercise is not only what you enjoy doing but also something that really leaves you feeling good. Use it or loose it, muscles quickly loose strength with disuse.

Exercise widens the arteries and blood circulation improves. Our muscles become efficient and we feel more fit. Thus, exercise improves muscle fitness which in turn will metabolize the food we eat more efficiently avoiding obesity.

Exercise during Pregnancy and after Childbirth

Exercise during pregnancy and after childbirth is very important.

On the advice of the doctor, a routine programme of regular exercise should be made. Exercise should be done first thing in the morning when one has lots of energy. In the western countries, classes and exercise routines are conducted in the antenatal clinics meant to strengthen abdominal & pelvic muscles. Vigorous exercise is not allowed during pregnancy, but moderate exercise such as walking, stretching of the arms, sweeping the floor helps in strengthening and relaxing perennial muscles which makes normal delivery easier. Even after delivery some simple exercise should be done to tone up the muscles of the body.

Healthy Eating

Important constituents of food include: Carbohydrates, fats, vitamins, protein, iron, calcium and salt. A healthy diet consists of all there in fixed proportions.

A healthy diet means healthy eating, that gives energy and vitality and supplies everything our body needs. Nutritious food include, bread, pulses, fruits, vegetables, meat, milk and water. Vitamin B is present in milk, meat, fish, eggs, butter, chicken, vegetables, fruits and curd. Carbohydrates are found in bread, potatoes, rice, cereals, plantains. Half of our intake of calories should consist of carbohydrates as they tend to cause weight gain are needed to maintain a healthy digestive system. They are found in vegetables, fruits, pulses, grains.

Fat intake according to WHO chart recommendation should not exceed one-third of our daily calories. Proteins are found in pulses, meat, chicken, fish, etc. Protein is necessary to build our body and later to repair wear and tear.

Vitamins

Our bodies are unable to produce them at all or in sufficient quantities. They are needed for growth and repair of the tissues.

There are two groups of vitamins— water soluble are B and C and fat soluble are A,D,E and K. Vitamins B and C are lost in cooking. Fruits and vegetables are therefore best sources of these vitamins.

Those who take a balanced diet of rice, milk, fruit, vegetables, meat, poultry, fish and pulse don't need vitamin supplements.

Salt

Salt is also essential for our bodies. Supplies iodine to our body.

Iron

Iron is particularly needed during pregnancy and is present in meat, vegetables, pulses, milk and grain.

Calcium

It is of importance in building and maintaining a healthy body. Loss of calcium leads to osteoporosis or brittle bones by which there can be fractures of bones on falling particularly at menopause and at the old age.

There are ways in which one can gradually establish a healthy eating pattern for oneself and the whole family rather than a revolution one week and relapse the next. Of all the meals we take, breakfast is the most important and essential. There is a long interval after dinner at night and the day ahead is full of activity and so to get energy, it is important to have proper breakfast. It is much more important for a pregnant woman.

Stress

Stress is very difficult to define and is imperfectly understood. Some doctors have defined it as 'the rate of wear and tear of the body and mind'.

When there is stress a person's blood pressure rises, the heart rate tends to change, sweating increases, mouth dries up, etc. Level of stress tends to correlate with duration and uncertainty which can magnify the stress response. The relationship between stress and all its symptoms can be complex and interactional. Example of this relationship is that stress can cause disturbed sleep and disturbed sleep can cause stress.

We live in an age where the pace of life seems to be accelerating all the time. Women are under stress throughout their lives. A girl during her childhood is frustrated as she is treated as a second rate member of the family and develops inferiority complex leading to stress. As she becomes a woman the anxiety of her parents regarding her marriage continues the stressful life. After marriage she is transplanted to an alien family with a different life-style than at her parents' house and adaptation to it adds to her stress. Impending motherhood though a natural and physiological event is a period of stress. As a mother nurturing the babies, their teething troubles, etc., are very stressful. For a working woman conditions between the demands of the family and her job are a regular source of frustration leading to stress.

The life they lead is just like the walk on a tight rope or balancing act. They feel guilty that they are not putting more of their time into motherhood and family, on account of their total commitment to their jobs, which feeling quite often affects their efficiency in their jobs and results in stress.

Caring for children may be physically demanding but it has its beneficial side. When youngsters become teenagers, to manage them is a psychological strain and yet parents miss them. Women always have to adjust and do not know how to deal with stress.

An unhealthy lifestyle is more stressful than a healthy one. Indulgence in too much of coffee or tea, smoking and drinking alcohol, also cause stress. One must examine reasons of stress in one's life and then see which one's you can eliminate or control. We have to develop a rapport with family members as they can give help and support whenever needed. A problem shared with family and friends is always better in order to reduce stress.

During the ageing years in particular, one must develop some kind of hobby, for example, reading, gardening or social work. This is the age when with loss of working, authority, fear of illness and death causes stress. There are various therapies and relaxation techniques, but the best is transcendental meditation as proved by research.

Counselling or Psychotherapy

It can help to discover the area in your lifestyle that is causing stress and changing them and coping with them.

A good night's sleep is an excellent antidote to stress, but it can be a casualty when stress sets in.

Hints when to rush to hospital due to Gynaecological Disorders

1. Acute pain in the abdomen, vomiting and collapse rush to a hospital (Ectopic pregnancy, twisting of the ovarian cyst, Appendicitis, etc.).
2. Bleeding per vaginium with or without pregnancy and after delivery or perperium.
3. Pure watery discharge per vaginium during pregnancy.
4. Pregnancy with convulsions and coma (Eclimpsia).

5. Excessive bleeding after the intercourse.
6. Injury (accidental) to the private parts
7. Sudden dimness of vision during pregnancy (Toximia).

When to Contact a Doctor

1. Contact bleeding (bleeding per vaginum during coitus).
2. Bleeding per vaginum after menopause.
3. Gastro intestinal disturbances.
4. If no menses even after the age of 17 years.
5. If menses continuing after the age of 55 years.
6. Lump in breast.
7. Stained discharge from the nipple (Breast cancer).
8. Stoppage of foetel movement during last two months of pregnancy.
9. Excessive vomiting during pregnancy.
10. Retention of urine.
11. Sudden loss of weight.
12. Jaundice.

55

YOGA

Dr. Vatsala Samant

In India the principles of yoga were laid down some 2000 years ago and are regarded as complete philosophy of life. Several different types of yoga have developed over the centuries. Yoga means "union". Hatha Yoga means self-discipline. There are various Asanas (postures) in yoga. There should be no excessive physical strain. It requires 10-15 minutes, once or twice a day and can be practiced by children and the aged people provided their health is sound.

It is advisable to start with a teacher and ensure that your bowels and bladder are empty. Yogic exercises should be done on an empty stomach and after a bath. Do not begin yoga if you have any disabilities or if you are under medical treatment.

Yoga

Tenacity is gained by stretching in various yoga postures or 'Asanas' two minutes at a time, while calmness comes with quiet consistent breathing and expansion of the wings. Pranayam yoga is a technique ideally suited to prevent physical and mental illness and to protect the body generally developing an inevitable sense of self-reliance and assurance. Yoga is a timeless pragmatic science evolved over thousands of years dealing with the physical, moral, mental, spiritual well-being of man as a whole. Asana or postures, bring steadiness in health and lightness to the limbs. A steady and pleasant posture produces mental equilibrium, they are not merely gymnastic exercises. A few things are required to perform, i.e., a clean place, a blanket and determination and no big fields as in other exercises and they are not expensive. One can do it alone and the equipment are one's limbs. They reduce fatigue and soothe the nerves and train and discipline the mind.

Pranayam: The word is derived from Prana which means length, expansion, stretching or Yama means breathing, respiratory, life, vitality, restraint and so pranayam means extension of breathing and its control or science of breathing.

Hints and cautions taken to practise yoga

1. Bladder and rectum should be empty.
2. Bath before and 15 minutes after yoga.
3. Empty stomach.
4. Time early morning and late evening.
5. Have place, airy, clean and free from noise.
6. No yoga after being in sun for several hours.
7. No extra strain.
8. Breath through nostrils.
9. To remove the fatigue lie down for sometime.
10. Avoid asanas during menses.

Pregnancy. All the asanas can be practised during the first three months of pregnancy. All the standing poses and the forward bending asanas may be done with mild movements, so that no pressure is felt in the abdomen. Certain asanas may be practised throughout pregnancy. To strengthen the pelvic muscles, reduce the labour pains. Pranayam may be practised throughout pregnancy as regular deep breathing will help considerably during labour. After delivery no 'Yogasanas' for a month, after that they can be practised mildly after three months.

How to Relax

Lying down on the ground like a corpse is called Shavasana. It removes fatigue and gives rest to the mind. Think of tension draining away like a dangerous poison from the muscles and body parts.

Conclusion

Yoga improves health and increases vitality along with inducing psycho-physical poise and relaxation. Relaxation of a profound quality is the greatest benefit that yoga offers to its European and American practitioners.

The pulls and pressures of today, destroy health and happiness through what are known as the 'stress diseases' and tensions within the psyche. Nothing like countering stress with the body's own defences! It is here primarily that yoga has proved so effective and so valuable for today's men and women.

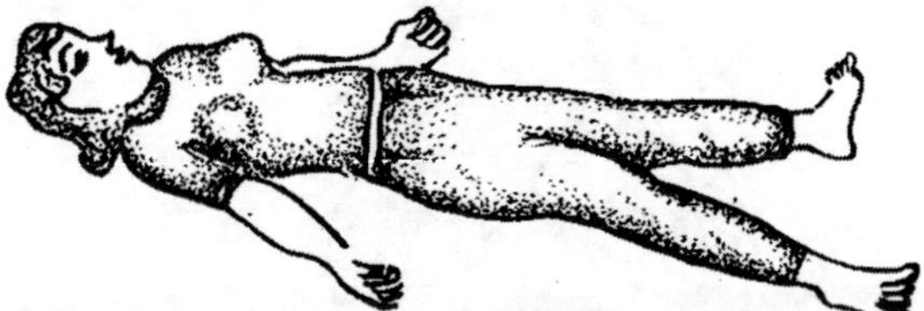

Shavasana

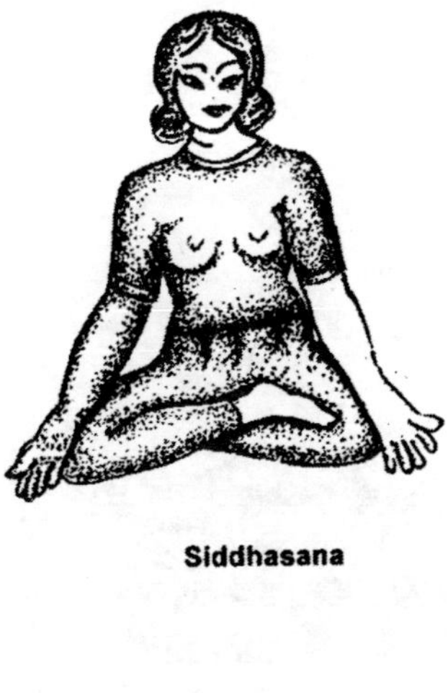

Siddhasana

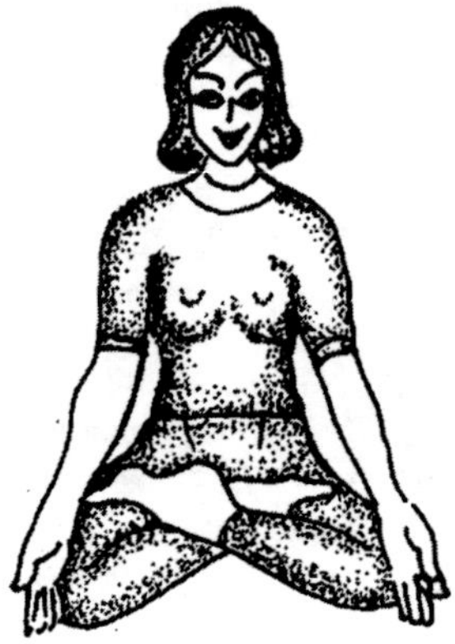

Padmasan

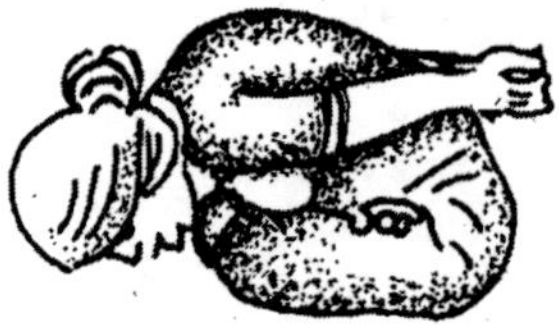

Yogasana

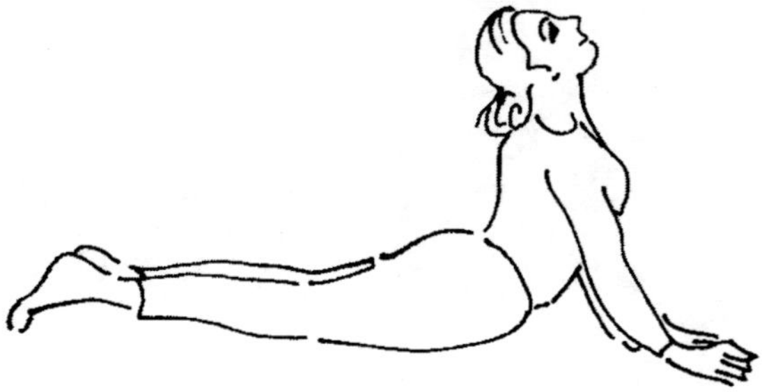

Bhujangasan

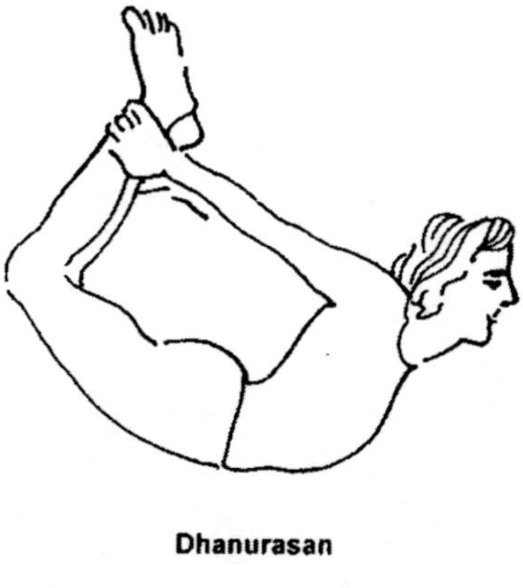

Dhanurasan

56

PHYSIOTHERAPY

Dr. Vatsala Samant

Physiotherapy is treatment of disease, injury or weakness in the joints or muscles by exercises, massage and the use of light, heat, etc.

During pregnancy there are various physical changes. Joints become loose, muscles are stretched, fat accumulates and so the weight is increased, etc. These changes lead to fatigue, changes in walking, sitting, lifting and even in breathing.

Labour is strenuous, exhausting and painful.

Throughout pregnancy during antenatal period certain exercises are taught. Antenatal exercises and relaxation methods lessons the strain during labour and makes labour easier.

Again in postnatal period getting the mother's abdominal muscles intact and getting back to her previous shape are taught by special type of exercises. This is what physiotherapy does—strengthens and relaxes joints and muscles and makes the mother fit.

Physiotherapy is of great help in restoring the pelvic floor muscles which surrounds the anus, vagina and urethra. Weakening of these during childbirth can give rise to incontinuance of urine and prolaps of the uterus.

Weakened abdominal muscles often cause backache. Hernia is caused by a swelling caused by the part of the bowl being pushed through a weak point of the wall of the abdomen. The object of physiotherapy is to lessen pregnancy discomforts, make labour easier and get back to normal shape in the post-natal period.

Physiotherapists should teach would be mothers and new mothers these special exercises.

57

ACUPUNCTURE

Dr. Vatsala Samant

A method to treat an illness or to anaesthetise a part of the body by putting the tips of a silver alloy or stainless steel needles into certain areas of the patient's skin and then vibrating them. The technique was first described by Chinese writers 4500 years ago. It is practised in India now and some of the allopathic doctors have taken training in this type of therapy and are practising the same.

Acupuncturists claim that this technique can alleviate or cure physical and mental ailments such as migraine, ulcers and digestive disorders, arthritis, asthma, depression and anxiety. They also stress that it should be continued with other forms of treatment, massage, hydrotherapy, diet control and exercises programme.

Acupuncture when tries on an expectant mother to reduce labour pains did not have any result.

58

BACKACHE

Dr. Vatsala Samant

Low backache affects women more than men. This can be explained by the fact that the female muscles and supports of the pelvics are not so strong as those of men. Backache in women exposed to the stress of pregnancy and pain, is worse before menses and quite often dates from pregnancy, labour and purperium. She is exposed to the nervous and emotional stress of motherhood and has inadequate rest and even sleep.

Gynaecological causes are displacement of the uterus, descent of the uterus or prolapse, infection of the pelvic organs, tumours of the uterus and ovary.

Extra genital causes are muscular or vertebral diseases, urinary trouble, arthritis or spondylitis.

Psychological Factors

In the majority of cases a gross reason is not found and the patient goes from one doctor to the other and finds no relief. Many sufferers of backache are of a complaining, and over anxious disposition. X-ray of the pelvics, vertebral column are a must for backache before naming it as psychological. Management of low backache is to find out the cause and its treatment. When no cause is found, reassurance and understanding; correction of the posture and organising life to provide interest is suggested I recommended.

Genital Prolapse

Downward descent of the uterus in the vagina is known as prolapse and is a very disabling condition.

Causes

Uterus and vagina are supported by pelvic muscles and

ligaments and correct abdominal pressure. Sometime there is a congenital weakness of these structures or the weakness is caused by childbirth injury. Chronic cough or fluid in the abdominal cavity increases intraabdominal pressure and causes descent of the uterus.

Ageing is another important factor to loosen the support and cause the descent of the uterus.

Treatment

If prolapse is of a minor degree, and if the patient is young, exercises to strengthen pelvic muscles are useful. Formerly ring pessary used to be inserted in the vagina to give support to the uterus. It used to cause infection and cases have been reported where the patient has forgotten about the pessary which became calcified causing more damage on removal of the pessary. Where there is recurrence, surgery is the final treatment. In young patients plastic supporting operation is done preserving uterus and enabling patient to have children, in old people particularly when the whole uterus is out, removal of the uterus without opening the abdomen is done.

59

INTERSEX

Dr. Vatsala Samant

It is a condition of imperfect sexual differentiation into either a male or female.

No human being is completely male or female as each contains rudimentary apparatus of the other. Many men are slightly effeminate and many women masculine in bearing and outlook, intersexuality can be physical or psychological or both.

Hermophrodite Eunuchs

They possess reproductive organs of both the sexes, ovary as well as testicles.

There are various types of intersexual beings. The earlier in life these errors are recognized and treated, better are the prospects for the individual to find a satisfactory place in society. These days it is in vogue to have operations for sex changes.

Sex is determined by chromozome studies. Parents of the child or patient, if adult, has to decide which sex, male or female is to be adopted permanently by the individual is concerned.

Hirsuitism

Slight hair on the upper lip, arms and legs is as much a female as a male characteristic. Some women can have hair on the chest and breasts. More important signs of masculinity are hair on beard area, legs, eyebrows extending over the bridge of the nose, nostrils and ears and baldness of the scalp.

Hirsuitism can be a sign of masculinizing tumours of the ovary and other ductless glands, but there are other signs also present.

Treatment

Cosmetics are indicated mainly in cases of simple hirsuitism. If the hair growth is slight nothing more than bleaching or application of depilatory wax is required.

60

HYSTERIA

Dr. Vatsala Samant

This is a condition in which the patient displays unusual behaviour generally to attract attention or to avoid unpleasant situation. It can be due to stress in an immature person who is vulnerable to suggestion. It is more common in women particularly in teenage girls.

Symptoms

Almost any symptoms can be produced by the hysteric persons ranging from pain, paralysis, convulsions, unconsciousness, etc. Cause is not known.

Treatment

Resolve the conflict and the cause of anxiety. Be firm and provide reassurance with minimum fuss. I have had cases of hysteric young girls showing all sorts of symptoms, counselling is the best way to cure them.

Hysteria is not a disease, but the patient particularly women show certain symptoms of some diseases, but there are no signs. I have had cases where the parents have brought their teenager school going girls complaining of acute pain in the stomach and fernity often and on quite often I have found that the cause of this behaviour is frustration, inability to study, etc. Generally another cause of Hysteria is infertility and to attract the attention of the family members. Sometime they act if uncessciousness and convulsion is so dramatic that even, a doctor is deceived.

The cause of Hysteria has to be investigated by counselling.

61

DIABETES

Dr. Sarita Bajaj, Ph.D.

What is Diabetes?

The disease diabetes whose name is derived from the Greek word meaning "Siphon" was known to ancient physicians. However, one of the first recorded references to diabetes is in the *Papyrus* discovered by Ebers in the tomb of Thebes in Egypt in 1862. Said to have been written in about 1500 BC, it was and is, the oldest book of any kind. Diabetes occurs either because of a lack of insulin or because of the presence of factors that oppose the action of insulin. The result of insufficient action of insulin is an increase in blood glucose concentration (hyperglycemia). Many other metabolic abnormalities occur, notably an increase in ketone bodies in the blood when there is a severe lack of insulin.

Diagnosis

The diagnosis of diabetes must always be established by measuring blood glucose concentration, although glycosuria usually (though not always) indicates disease.

Criteria for diagnosis are:

1. Symptoms of diabetes plus casual (i.e. at any time of day without regard to time since last meal) plasma glucose concentration $\geq$ 200 mg /dl.
2. Fasting plasma glucose (FPG) > 126 mg/dl.
3. 2 hours plasma glucose of > 200 mg/dl.

These criteria should be confirmed by repeat testing on a different day.

Common Mistakes in Diagnosis

1. Diagnosis and treatment of diabetes on detection of urine glucose alone.
2. Diagnosis by blood glucose strip alone (Glucometer). This is not reliable enough to make a lifelong diagnosis.
3. Requesting a blood test after intake of glucose (glucose tolerance test) when the diagnosis is already confirmed.

Types of Diabetes

The vast majority of cases of diabetics fall into two categories. In one category (type 1 or insulin dependent diabetes) the cause is an absolute deficiency of insulin secretion. Type 1 diabetics need insulin forever. In the other category (type 2 or non-insulin dependent diabetes), the cause is a combination of resistance to insulin action and an inadequate compensatory insulin secretory response. In the latter category, a degree of hyperglycemia sufficient to cause pathologic and functional changes in target tissues, but without clinical symptoms may be present for a long period of time (up to 12 years) before diabetes is detected. During this asymptomatic period, it is possible to demonstrate an abnormality in carbohydrate metabolism by measurement of plasma glucose in the fasting state or after a challenge with an oral glucose load. Type 2 diabetics may need insulin for control when oral drugs fail to do so.

Type 1 diabetes is auto immune in origin, whereas type 2 is multifactorial. Two factors stand out distinctly in its causation:

1. Genetic factors
2. Environmental factors

The interaction of the genetic factors with the various environmental factors culminates in the final development of the disease. It is obvious that while the genetic factors cannot be modified after birth, the environmental factors can definitely be influenced to a great extent.

Risks of Inheriting Diabetes

For type 1 diabetes

Relative of proband

Parent	3%
Child	6%

With affected father	8%
With affected mother	3%
Sibling	5%
Identical twin	33%

Individuals at increased risk to develop type 1 diabetes (in decreasing order)

1. Monozygotic twin of type 1 diabetic
2. Sibling of a type 1 diabetic
3. Offspring of a type 1 diabetic

For Type 2 Diabetes

If someone in the family has diabetes	20%
If one parent has diabetes	40%
If one parent has diabetes and the other parent is from a diabetic family	70%
If both parents have diabetes	99%

Clearly inheritance is more important in type 2 diabetes.

Individuals at increased risk to develop type 2 diabetes (in decreasing order)

1. Monozygotic twin of type 2 diabetic
2. Other first degree relatives of a type 2 diabetic
   (a) Sibling (especially if both parents are diabetic)
   (b) Parent
   (c) Offspring
3. Obese individuals
4. Mother who has delivered a baby > 4.5 kg. weight

Who Should be Screened?

1. Persons with a family history of diabetes
2. Persons who are markedly obese
3. Persons with high blood pressure
4. Persons with an abnormal lipid profile

5. Women with a bad obstetric history—recurrent stillbirths, abortions, delivering malformed babies, elderly women, women with a large parity and those who have delivered large babies.

6. All pregnant women

7. Patients with recurrent genital, urinary tract or skin infections

8. Patients with otherwise unexplained

— Neuropathy

— Atherosclerosis

— Coronary artery disease

— Peripheral vessel disease

— Retinopathy

— Nephropathy

— All pre-operative patients

9. Testing for diabetes should be considered in all individuals at age 45 years and above and, if normal, it should be repeated at 3-year intervals.

Presentation, Symptoms and Signs

Thirst, tiredness, genital itching, passing excessive urine, and weight loss despite excessive hunger are the familiar symptoms of diabetes. Why then is the diagnosis so often missed?

Patients do not, of course, always describe their symptoms in the clearest possible terms, or else their complaints may occur only as an indirect consequence of the more common features. Many patients describe dry mouth rather than thirst and are then investigated for dysphagia. Frequency is often treated blindly with antibiotics; children may start bedwetting and incontinence may be a manifestation in elderly people; and the true diagnosis is overlooked. Complex urological investigations are sometimes performed before the urine is tested. Some diabetic patients present chiefly with weight loss (despite an increased appetite), but even then the diagnosis is sometimes missed. Perhaps weakness, tiredness, and lethargy, which may be the dominant symptoms, are the most commonly misinterpreted. Tonics and vitamins are sometimes given as the symptoms worsen.

Deteriorating vision is not uncommon as a presentation, due either to a change of refraction causing myopia or to the early development of retinopathy. Foot ulceration or sepsis in older patients brings them to accident and emergency departments and is nearly always due to diabetes. Occasionally neuritis is the presenting symptom, causing exquisite pain in the feet, thighs or trunk.

Some older men are first aware of diabetes when they notice white spots on their trousers. In hot climates drops of sugary urine attract an interested population of ants. Symptoms are similar in the two types of diabetes (types 1 and 2), but they vary in their intensity. The presentation is most typical and the symptoms develop most rapidly in patients with type 1 diabetes. Symptomatic type 2 diabetics represent the tip of an iceberg, the majority being asymptomatic. It is common to disbelieve a raised blood glucose report in the absence of symptoms, but it must be confirmed by a repeat test on a subsequent day and if still abnormal, be appropriately treated irrespective of symptoms.

The diagnosis of diabetes should no longer be missed. New patients attending their doctor, whether their family doctor or at a hospital outpatient clinic, should have a blood glucose measurement or at the very least a urine test especially if their symptoms are unexplained.

Prevalence

Type 1 diabetes constitutes only 2 per cent of diabetes. The remaining (98 per cent) have type 2 diabetes. The prevalence of diabetes differs widely for different ethnic groups and countries. For example, it can range from <3 per cent among rural communities in developing countries to almost 50 per cent in Pima Indians in the USA.

Though the incidence of diabetes is increasing worldwide, the dubious distinction of being the country with the largest number of diabetic individuals and the greatest predicted increase in the prevalence of diabetes (200 per cent between 1995 and 2005), lies with India.

While the prevalence of diabetes in rural Indians remains low (2-5 per cent), in urban areas it has risen to 10-20 per cent. Type 2 diabetes affects Indians at a younger age than in the west. Thus, it affects patients during their most productive years and also increases the chances that chronic complications may ensue. Indian type 2 patients are in general far less obese than their western counterparts. Type 2 diabetes has reached epidemic proportions in Indians. An interplay of environmental factors as well as genetic predisposition is probably responsible. Increasing urbanization and adoption of a westernized lifestyle with changes in diet as well as reduced physical activity are likely causes. A genetic predisposition is evident from the strong familial aggregation. The predisposing genes are, however not yet known.

Complications of Diabetes

Patients with longstanding diabetes may develop complications affecting the eyes, kidneys, nerves, heart, and blood vessels. Long-term complications of diabetes include: retinopathy with potential loss of vision, nephropathy leading to renal failure, peripheral neuropathy with risk of foot ulcers and amputation and autonomic neuropathy causing gastrointestinal, genitourinary, and cardiovascular symptoms and sexual dysfunction. Patients with diabetes have an increased incidence of atherosclerotic, cardiovascular, peripheral vascular, and cerebrovascular disease. Hypertension, abnormalities of lipoprotein metabolism, and periodontal disease are often found in people with diabetes. The emotional and social impact of therapy may cause significant psychosocial dysfunction in patients and their families.

Coronary artery disease (angina, myocardial infraction) and stroke are more common in diabetics.

Investigations to be Performed at Regular Intervals

(1) Fasting and Post Prandial blood glucose

(2) Kidney tests : Microalbuminuria

Complete urine examination

Serum urea and creatinine

(3) Eye examination : Ophthalmoscopy

(4) Electrocardiogram

(5) Complete lipid profile

(6) Glycosylated haemoglobin (HbA_1c)

Treatment and Prevention

There is no cure for diabetes in any science, today. The aims of treatment are, first, to save life and alleviate symptoms, and secondly, to achieve the best possible control of diabetes with blood glucose concentrations as near normal as possible to minimize long-term complications. Control is achieved by:

(i) Diet and exercise alone

(ii) Diet, exercise and oral drugs

(iii) Diet, exercise and insulin

Diet and exercise are the cornerstones on which the management of diabetes rests.

There is no substitute. Decision regarding drug, insulin therapy should be taken by the consultant endocrinologist. Other important aims in mangement include control of weight and elimination of risk factors, notably hypertension, smoking, and hazards to the feet.

Primary prevention can be achieved by identifying high risk subjects at an early stage and imparting appropriate health education to them and the community. Fasting hyperglycemia can be prevented in 90 per cent of individuals who are at risk of developing it by maintaining ideal body weight throughout a lifetime or losing excess body weight. All it takes is a 30 minute walk a day! Secondary prevention aims at early diagnosis and appropriate treatment of the disease to reduce morbidity and mortality and rehabilitation of those physically handicapped due to the disease.

There are currently 20 million type 2 diabetics in India, and these will increase to 57 million in the next 25 years. There is an urgent need to put into place programmes which will prevent the development of diabetes in susceptible individuals, provide diabetes education to healthcare professionals, and improve patient care so that chronic complications of diabetes are reduced. Such a diabetes prevention and control programme has, unfortunately, not yet been formulated at the national level.

62

FIBROMYALGIA

Dr. Vatsala Samant

Fibromyalgia or FM is a common and disabling disorder affecting women more than men and diagnosis is often missed. FM is not new, only the name is. Since the physicians during the ninteenth century have recognized it and written about a condition involving sleep, fatigue, stiffness, and pain for which there is little or no diagnostic explanation and called it muscular rheumatism.

FM patients usually ache all over, sleep poorly, are stiff on walking, and are tired all day. They are prone to headache, memory, concentration problems, dizziness, numbness, tingling, itching, fluid retension, abdominal or pelvic pain and diarrhoea. It often runs in the families suggesting an inherited predisposition.

It may be dormant until triggered by an injury stress or sleep disturbances. However no inflammation or arthritis has been found and it is believed that depression, anxiety, when present are more often the result than the cause of FM. There is evidence that FM is due to an abnormal brain waves, in deep sleep. Abnormal brain waves have been found in many patients of FM. FM like symptoms can be produced in normal volunteers by depriving deep sleep for a few days. Growth hormone which maintains good muscle and soft tissue healthy is produced in deep sleep and is found to be low in FM patients.

Exercise is supposed to increase production of the growth hormone. Taking medicines by itself has relatively little effect on FM symptoms. Successful treatment requires active involvement of the patient in his/her case including medication to improve regular sleep hours, and adequate amount of nutrition, etc.

There are other several alternative remedies such as herbal, transcendental meditation. FM sufferers do not elicit sympathy and support they deserve from family, friends and employers because of the lack of outward evidence of disease. They have been told by their physicians that there is nothing wrong with them or it is all in their head which is demoralizing but nobody knows the whole truth or the cause of FM.

There is a legend about four blind men and the elephant, each had his hand on a different part of the animal and they were arguing that the animal was like the part of the body which they were holding. One holding the tail said it was a rope. Another holding the leg said it was a tree and third one touching the body said it was a wall. Another holding its ear said it was like a fan. Each had a part of the truth but none could see the whole animal. FM is lot like that elephant as described by the blind men. FM is classified as a syndrome rather than a disease because disease is a condition that has a known cause and can be identified by one or other set of laboratory tests which unfortunately appear to be all normal in FM cases.

Living well with FM means finding the right balance of sleep, exercise, nutrition, psychological or spiritual well-being. One should try to change FM from something disabling to something manageable.

Fibromayalgia in Children

Until recently FM was considered an adult syndrome but studies have shown that it can affect children also. FM in children often starts with a flue like illness from which the child seems never to recover fully. FM simply comes in gradually without any precipitating event in children before puberty. One should suspect FM in a child who sleeps restlessly, has a difficult time getting up out of bed in the morning. A child who learns good nutritional habits early in life, grows accutomed to going to bed at the same time every night and encouraged to take part in a suitable exercise programme will be equipped to avoid FM flareups throughout life.

I am a patient suffering from FM. It is a terrible syndrome to have, since few people have knowledge of it. This is what makes it very difficult to deal with this situation. Lack of knowledge.

About 5-6 years back I noticed a change in my pain. I have always suffered from pain since the age of 20. At that time All India Medical Institute of Sciences had diagnosed me with rheumatoid arthritis. It started with my small joints and over the years encroached my body. Some years back I thought I had gone into remission, I was totally relieved of my pain. Soon thereafter I fell ill with fever. It was a low grade fever, which was earlier described as thyphoid and almost a year later with tuberculosis.

During this time I noticed a change in my attitude and pain. My bones no longer hurt it was a muscular pain. The areas were specified, my chest muscles, upper arms, lower hips and my shoulders. The doctors kept pacifying me that it was my arthritis and that my muscles and tissues were involved. I learned to live with it since there was nothing I could do. Along with all of this my emotions had taken a change which I was unable to answer. Since I could not express myself, I started withdrawing. The night before I use to be in perfect health and in the morning I found it difficult to function, let alone get out of bed. Since my understanding was nil on this, I found it difficult to communicate, when I was asked what is the matter with me, and that is the reason for my withdrawal. It was probably the worst period in my life. I did not associate with anyone, to the extent that I started avoiding my children. It hurt terribly. During this time my sleep pattern changed and I found it very difficult to fall asleep. The longest has been 13 consecutive nights of no sleep. By this time my whole body was in tremors, but there was no tiredness from lack of sleep. I functioned normally except for the pain, which was there almost everyday, sometimes more and sometimes bearable. I was given valium tablets as well as valium injections so that I could get some rest, but nothing helped. I still did not sleep. Finally I was given a medication that did help me to sleep and the tremors disappeared. I felt so relaxed and releived. Within a few days it was back to sleepness nights.

Months later a doctor I saw in America gave me an article to read out of a medical journal. Upon reading it I will say that I was half cured. The article was as if I had written my own story. I felt that I am not imagining it and it is something that others have also. That was the day my treatment started. I had been told many a times by friends and family that I should see a psychiatrist.

The medication was anti-depressants (Amitryptheline). This drug builds up the seretonin level in your brain which enables you to sleep, so when you wake up the next morning you have enough energy to fight the fatigue.

You see, fatigue takes over and all your muscles go into a spasm. Since one has muscles everywhere, your eyes don't open or your vision is not clear. There is difficulty in breathing since the muscles around your lungs don't work, similarly the rest of the body. All you can do is rest. Since any type of movement is almost impossible this is the only thing one can resort to. Usually the next day it is as though nothing has happened.

It is said that an injury is often responsible for the onset of Fibromyalgia. I did have an injury that I can relate to. At the age of 18 I fell down a flight of staires and broke my tailbone, any a few later it broke again at the same spot.

What I found most distressing was the fact that no one seem to understand what I was going through. Educating the ones who my life was associated with was my major concern, but you cannot do this without the willingness of the individual involved.

First I educated myself, through books, support groups, and collecting information from professionals who were aware of this problem.

For my own sanity I had to inform others I dealt with on a day to day basis about my problem. I thank God that, that has been taken care of.

I have over the years changed many drugs under the supervision of doctors. Some have had bad side effects on me unabling me to continue with it.

My symptoms keep changing, never has the pain disappeared though. It may have gotten worse, but I have learnt to live with it and through means of educating myself I have been a great source of strength to myself.

My memory fails me. My body does not carry out the duties that I would like for it to do, my thoughts and feelings are very different at times to the person I once was. I have had to make many adjustments and I continue to do so almost everyday. I plan everything a few days in advance, since I do not know what tomorrow will be like for me. I look more than healthy but my system has disowned me. I still have lots to be grateful for, seeing others in misery makes feel blessed that I do have some good days, and it is not life threatening, even if I cannot start my days in the mornings.

My children, husband and my family have now upon understanding, given me more support than I could have dreamt of. Though it is never enough when the pain takes over.

I still go into deep depressions and try to fight it for the sake of those around me, so as not to alarm them. But most of the time I am putting up a brave front and it exhausts me. I sincerely hope that anyone who is suffering from this has gained some strength from this article. I know I have from reading others experiences. Knowing that is it not imaginary and that I am not the only one.

I wish to help anyone who needs my support.

Rubina Shervani.

63

MALARIA

Dr. Vatsala Samant

India was virtually free of malaria in the 1960s as a result of widespread use of DDT. Now malaria is again the biggest public health problem contributing to 39 per cent of all reported cases outside Africa. If not properly diagnosed by doctors, patients may die within three days. Eradication, the dogma of 1966, is no longer considered to be realistic and the goal now is to promote early diagnosis, build and initiate a range of flexible community based efforts to the vector mosquitoes, to mobilize local resources to fight it. Now there are very few tools to control malaria. The parasite adapts to new drugs very fast. After all the microbes fight for their survival as well as people. The parasite develops resistance when it encounters a concentration of the drug that is not potent to kill it and this happens when patients fail to take the full course of the drug that is prescribed for the treatment or when drugs are used indiscriminately as prophylaxis. What is needed is improved health care facilities, more focus on spraying campaigns and neighbourhood cleanliness programmes to eliminate breeding places for the mosquitoes and better environmental management. Malaria must become everybody's problem.

Dengue

It is a common viral disease of the tropics and subtropics. It is transmitted to man by a bite from the infected mosquitol. The incubation period is 5 to 8 days. Dengue symptoms come on suddenly. There is pain in the joints, muscles, a high fever, backache and a widespread skin rash. Treatment is to rush the patient to the doctor. The only preventive measure is avoiding mosquitoe bites.

64

ANAEMIA

Dr. Vatsala Samant

Anaemia is defined as reduction in the haemoglobin mass that circulates in our blood below the critical level. The normal concentration varies between men and women, but the average in women is 12-14 per cent. Anaemia is very common in India and particularly in pregnant women. Data suggests that about half of the pregnant women and one-third of the non-pregnant in the world suffer from nutritional anaemia. Anaemia particularly during pregnancy is emerging, as number one health problem, and is the main cause of maternal morbidity and mortality. It can cause abortion, premature and low weight babies.

Causes of Anaemia

The main cause is nutritional deficiency, bleeding hemolysis as happens in malaria but the most important is iron and folate deficiency. Thalassemia a congenital disorder in which a person is born with less HB is common in some parts of India. Parasitic infestation particularly hookworm is another cause of anaemia, because nutritional anaemia is the most common cause. Iron stores at birth are minimum in male and female at birth.

In India, there is a gender bias. The girl child receives inferior treatment from beginning and it is likely that high incidence of anaemia in Indian women is related to gender bias.

Diagnosis

There may be vague complaints like ill-health, fatigue, loss of appetite, breathlessness, exertion and palpitation. Examination reveals pallor, pale nails and tongue. HB estimation and complete blood tests such as RBC count, etc., confirm the diagnosis of anaemia.

Management

The average vegetarian diet contains very little iron and in India women enter pregnancy when they are already depleted of iron and so there is a need for routine administration of iron to pregnant women. It is advisable to build iron stores in all women even before they get married and conceive. Primary education is compulsory and if adolescent girls are provided iron supplements in their school with mid-day meals it may help building iron stores.

Treatment

Iron tablets by mouth or by injection if necessary, is a must depending on HB count. Folates vitamins are needed for maturation of RBC. They are present in liver, green vegetables, spinach, sweet potatoes, bananas, mangoes, etc. If they are boiled these vitamins are destroyed. Vit B_{12} is very useful, the main source of which is found in meat, fish, eggs and in milk.

Causes

Malaria is a major factor causing severe anaemia and as malaria is rampant in India malarial prophylaxis is of benefit in areas where it is endemic or seasonal.

Worm Infestation

Hookworm is an important cause of anaemia. They produce iron deficiency due to chronic blood loss in the digestive system, and thus they deplete iron stores. Stool examination can give the diagnosis.

As a preventive measure and also to prevent recurrence, patients should be advised to use footwear, improve sanitation, and personal hygiene and safe drinking water.

Hookworm eggs are found in the soil and people working in the fields barefooted get infected with these worms.

Comment

We have had cases with 2 to 4 gms HB in the last stage of prolonged labour at home delivery coming to us in a serious condition. They deliver with the help of forceps. In the 3rd stage there is always bleeding not very profound but enough for these anaemic patients to go into heart failure and succumb, before we could arrange blood transfusion. Even non-pregnant women coming for operation are found to be anaemic particularly middle-class women who are undernourished because they eat what remains after the children and family had their meals. HB estimation should be done. Anaemia in pregnancy could be avoided by proper pre-natal and post-natal care and by having correct nutrition and diet.

65

TUBERCULOSIS

Dr. Vatsala Samant

Recent studies have revealed the magnitude of the problem of TB which remains the biggest killer in the world as a single pathogen. It hits children as well as elderly people, but the worst affected are adults between 15 and 59 years of age. TB accounts for 26 per cent of all avoidable deaths in the Third World countries. There is an interaction between HIV and TB. The toll of TB is increasing in many countries, even then TB is curable even in the HIV infected patients. Proper diagnosis and adequate management of cases can stop the perpetuation and elimination of the disease. Almost all the patients with newly diagnosed TB can be cured if properly treated and many will die if not properly treated. TB is a challenging disease.

TB is an infectious disease and can affect any and every organ in our body, for example, brain (meningitis), intestines, bones, skin, lungs, reproductive organs, etc.

Causes

(1) From spitting or coughing of adults who have TB of the lung, TB bacilli are dropped and are forced in the air and are carried away in the air. In closed rooms, huts, the bacilli in the atmosphere of the room remain and every one sharing the room runs the risk of contacting TB. An infected mother is a danger to the suckling infant.

(2) From food or milk, cows are infected with Bovine TB which affects the udder of the cow and T. bacilli are found in the milk if the milk is not boiled. T bacilli reach the intestines and cause intestinal TB. From the intestine they travel to peritoneum and from there they infect the reproductive track. These bacilli can remain inactive for couple of years but they are alive and capable of multiplying and later on enter the bloodstream and affect any organ.

Symptoms

Symptoms depend upon the organs infected with TB. BCG is a vaccine consisting of live T. bacilli which have lost their virulence. These bacilli originally came from a strain of bovine TB grown for many years in the laboratory. BCG invigorates our body defence without itself causing damage. Following BCG vaccination T. bacilli may enter the body but in most cases the body's increased defence will control or kill the bacilli. The effect lasts for 15 years.

Prevention

Every newborn should be given BCG. Direct sunlight kills T. Bacilli in 5 minutes, therefore exposure to sunlight is a convenient and useful method. Paper handkerchiefs should be burnt as soon as possible after use by the TB patients.

Environmental Hygiene

The aim of environmental hygiene is to reduce the risk from sputum of undiagnosed patients, improve ventilation, improve nutrition particularly in poverty stricken population, examine relatives particularly those staying with TB patients and giving BCG vaccination to the inmates of the house. Promote healthy habit among people and informs people about the cleanliness.

Treatment

There are various kinds of anti TB. drugs and the treatment by drugs should be left upon the doctor. But the treatment should be continued as long as advised by the doctor and there should be no defaulting.

If the treatment is incomplete it will have a devastating effect. Tuberculosis can virtually always be cured and spread prevented.

Abdominal Tuberculosis

It is common amongst people who do not boil milk properly particularly in the rural area where cows milk is used. Cows suffer for Tuberculosis and the udders are affected, and Tubercular bacterias contaminate the milk and thus, intestine infection takes place. Signs and symptoms are intestinal upset diarrhoea. Loss of appetite, mild fever, loss of weight and bloating of the Abdomen due to Tubercular Abcities.There is palpapatin of the abdomen and lumps can be felt. Treatment of course is the same anti-tubercular.

Reproductive Tuberculosis is due to the spread of abdominal Tuberculosis from the peritourism or lenning of the abdomen to the fallopian tubes of the uterus and ovaries.

Tuberculosis Meningitis

Like cancer Tuberculosis affects all the systems and organs of the body. When affects central nervous system particularly menenges evening streath of the spinal cord the disease is known as meningitis. It can affect at any age but is common in children. Signs are high fever, muscular disturbance such as convulsions going on to coma if not detected. Diagnosis is based on teemper pueture and microscopic organism of cerebrospinal fluid. If diagnosed and treated early there is complete recovery. I have known the case of an old lady who went into convulsions and common with high fever tumber prenuter examination of the cerebrot spinal fluid was done which confirmed the diagnosis of Tubercular meningitis. Treatment was started and she recovered though if took about months because of her old ase, though a little bit of effect of the disease in her gait and memory is left which I am sure will disappear in due course of time.

66

HEPATITIS B

Dr. Vatsala Samant

Hepatitis is a disease that involves inflammation of the liver. There are two types of hepatitis, viral and toxic.

Hepatitis B

This is spherical, shelled virus with a double standard DNA as its genetic material. It requires a longer incubation period than type A with the period ranging from four to twenty-five weeks. The viroids are seen in large numbers in the bloodstream of affected people. The virus was once commonly transmitted through the transfusion of contaminated blood. Hence the name serum hepatitis and transfusion hepatitis. Nowadays techniques are available to check the blood for the virus before transfusion yet, infections do take place through improperly sterilized medical instruments. Medical personnel such as doctors and nurses are more at a risk of getting infected. Drug addicts who use needles are also a high risk group. Infection can also take place through sexual contact. Hepatitis B virus is carried in the blood of a recovered patient for years. They can transmit the disease even though they no longer suffer from it. Such people are called carriers. The virus is seen in the body fluids of the carriers such as saliva, sweat, and milk and this makes the person to person transmission quite likely. About 1 per cent of patients die from serums hepatitis.

Symptoms

Hepatitis involves the inflammation of the liver. The symptoms of this disease are: There is a preliminary stage characterised by fever, headache and loss of appetite. Then comes a stage of jaundice in which the yellowing of the skin, eyes and body cavities takes place because the blood contains too much of vilirubin, a constituent of bile. At the same time spleen and liver become tender and the appetite is almost completely lost. Nausea and vomiting are common. Urine becomes dark yellow. Jaundice lasts for two to five weeks and then disappears. A gradual recovery followers, unless there are some complications.

Precautionary measures against hepatitis B include checking of blood before transfusion, use of properly sterilized medical instruments and avoidance of close contact with the carriers. As far as treatment is concerned it should be left to the doctors.

67

OBESITY

Dr. Vatsala Samant

More females than males are overweight at any age, the frequency of overweight increases with age to a peak at 35 to 44 years in males and at age 55 to 64 in females. A number of factors including age, sex and physical activity influences the amount of body fat. At puberty there is a significant increase in the percentage of fat in females and fall in males.

Risks Related to Obesity

Obesity is a risk factor particularly in younger males who are substantially overweight. In older individuals those who are moderately overweight and in women the risk is less. The principle cause of mortality include diabeties melitus, hypertension and sudden death. In females there is an increased frequency of abnormal menstrual cycles with obesity. Return of menstrual regularity is often found with weight loss and increased fertility is possible. Pregnancy augments weight gain.

Causes (Etiology) of Obesity

(i) *Etiology.* Neuroendocrine disease such as pituitary and thyroid disfunctioning.

(ii) *Drug induced obesity.* Overzealous treatment of diabeties with insulin increases hunger and intake of food and if continued may increase obesity.

(iii) *Cortico Steroid therapy.* Dietary obesity, excessive consumption of sugar, sweetened beverages with prevalence of abundant varieties in cafeteria, may be dietary factors in the development of obesity.

(iv) *Genetic factor.* If both the parents are obese, 80 per cent offsprings will be obese. If only one parent is obese about 14 per cent of the offsprings will be obese. If none of the parent is obese obesity in the offsprings falls to 10 per cent.

Treatment of obesity

Calorie restriction. Calorie intake must be reduced. This requires a daily assessment of calorie requirements. Fasting may help.

Therefore obesity may be one of the manifestations of certain diseases such as diabeties, melitus, hypertension, heart disease or gallbladder stones.

All these diseases should be ruled out by proper tests, whether these disorders are present or not in the obese person he should be encouraged to loose weight by appropriate methods. These include diet, nutritional education, self-help, group behavioural changes, exercise, and physical activity.

Obesity

Obesity occurs more often in women than in men and usally starts in the middle years of life. Heredity is a possible cause. The most common offender lies in habits and cating-eating too much and moving around too little fails to consiene the caloric value.This lays up as fat

Since it is difficult for people to control their did they have recourse too sha methods and one of therapy is with cold water. Cold water steps up metabolism. Fat is consumed, digesting and absorb are improved thyroid, ovaries, pitutary which fat becoming glands are stimulated.

Among other factors related to obesity are frustation, unhappeners, nervous tension, etc.

As weight grow there is pain in the feet and knees. One can develop high blood pressure.

Psychological problems lead to eating and degging ones own grave.

Sweating causes dicongstion and stimulates digestion organs. and so hot water baths undues swealling.

Regular controlled exercise programme should be worked out on a daily bass, which burn calories. Dietary controls but not crash programme. One is fat in direct proportion to the fired you burn.

In getting rid of obesity, you need more than a desire.

68

SLEEP: A DIVINE GIFT

Dr. Vatsala Samant

Sleep is of great importance to mankind. Night is meant to sleep for human beings, animals and birds. Birds get into their nests. Flowers particularly lotus closes its petals only to smile and bow to the rising sun in the morning thus inviting everybody to wake up and start their daily chores. Generally we spend one-third of our life asleep. How well we sleep is a major determinant of how well we live. Sleep affects us as to how we feel both physically and mentally, how you behave, how well you can handle the ordinary stresses of life, how you get along with people and how productive and happy you are.

If you are not sleeping well you are cranky or depressed, accident-prone, a danger to yourself and others. You will find it difficult to think, to reason, to remember. Sleep depravation has been an effective weapon to torture prisoners and also to brain wash them. Lack of sleep harms your immune system and makes you vulnerable to the invasion of viruses and we are unable to fight them.

Individuals vary greatly in the amount of sleep they need. For an adult, average is between 7 to 8 hours, for some 5 to 6 hours is enough. But there is a great variation from person to person in the amount of sleep required. Infants need more sleep of almost 18 hours. The period of sleep becomes less and less as we grow up. The pattern of your needs vary from day to day as you reach adulthood. As you grow older, you tend to sleep more lightly at night and may nap during the day which can make one even more watchful at night.

Awake or asleep, your brain produces electrical currents shown as waves known as EEG, which can be measured and show the average activity of the brain or nerve cells. EEG is painless and shows how many times you wake up during the night and how much restful sleep you had. There are two kinds of sleep— Rapid eye movements (REM) and Nonrapid eye movements (NREM). Dream sleep is REM sleep. Our eyes move when we dream as if we are looking at something. Research has shown that psychological problems are built from lack of REM sleep. The important thing to remember about the duration of sleep is this, if you wake up feeling rested, if your alertness and energy during the day is satisfactory then you are getting enough of sleep. But if you wake up feeling deprived of sleep and drag through the day in an irritable fog, then you have sleep problem regardless of the number of hours you spend in bed with your eyes closed.

Sleep Disturbances

There is some evidence that sleep disturbances may be caused by an abnormality of deep sleep. It is during deep delta or deep sleep that the body does its repair work and replenishment. The hormone Somatostatin which is produced in deep sleep is vital for maintaining muscles and soft tissues in good health. This hormone is less in some diseases. If deep sleep is reduced over a long period of time, the body may have less ability to repair and replenish energy. Experiments on animals showed that destruction of the part of the brain that housed Seratonin contained in the nerve cells could produce total insomnia. Partial Serotonin damage to these area of the brain caused various variable decrease in sleep. This hormone is present in milk and so a warm cup of milk seems to help some individuals to sleep. Here are some tips to insure sleep.

Sleep as much as is needed to feel refreshed and healthy. A regular waking time in the morning strengthens circadian cycling and leads to regular times of sleep. Hunger may disturb sleep and so light snack before going to bed may help. Caffeine disturbs sleep so also tobacco. Use the bed only for sleeping. Do not sleep during the day.

Another cause of sleep disturbance is the bed mate snoring. Sugar also can make sleep elusive. Other elements that can disturb sleep included much light or noise in the room, poor ventilation, wrong kind of pillow and mattresses. Deep restful sleep is your best ally in fighting illness. Maintaining a regular schedule that allows sufficient sleep is necessary.

Night is meant for sleep but due to TV the lifestyle of our people has changed. Late nights, getting up late in the morning, just having a cup of coffee and rushing to the office is the routine today. This is the cause of heart disease, stroke and many other ailments. Regular exercise helps to sleep, so also soft music.

Insomnia

Insomnia is sleepless nights over a long period. The causes could be anxiety, depression or problems troubling a person. If one has difficulty in sleeping and one is not over estimating the amount of sleep you need, then the first step is to remove the problem which keeps you awake and try to develop relaxation techniques. Sleeping pills are no answer because they could add to the same problems and you can get addicted and immune to them, so avoid taking sleeping pills.

69

COUNSELLING: A THERAPY

Mitali Tandon

Counselling must have existed since the very beginning of human civilization. Man must have sought help, guidance, advice and comfort from family members, friends and close associates. Civilization is becoming more complex—the rapid advance of modern science and technology has not only led to tremendous progress but has also brought about a number of unprecedented problems. The disintegration of the joint family system has also given rise to one major problem—that of finding 'solace' from family members. With the continuous social changes, man now possesses a fantastic opportunity for self-determination to pursue unexplored avenues and for enjoying life to its fullest potential.

In such a transitional era, it is becoming more and more necessary for professional and scientific counselling to become a specialized job to help people. A professional counsellor realizes that the ultimate concern lies with the person who needs help to strengthen himself to cope with his problems.

Counselling concerns several vital problems. The first concerns family health and education. With the population explosion, there is an urgent need for women to be appropriately counselled regarding family health. Women have to learn to face the challenge of transitions in life situations. Women today have more avenues open to them. According to a leading psychologist, young women today have a conflict between their need for achievement and the need to conform to their female image—that of a wife, a daughter-in-law, a mother and so on. Such conflicts lead to negative emotional consequences. The role of the counsellor, therefore, would be to build self-confidence not merely at the intellectual level but also at the affective level. Counselling can also extend to middle aged women who find themselves left in a void, facing an identity crisis while their children are grown up and are preoccupied with their studies and other jobs. The mother is not needed—this creates a sense of emptiness in her and she can be counselled to occupy herself gainfully to her satisfaction. Early intervention of counsellors prevents such problems to become chronic.

Often, a counsellor's role is mistaken with that of a psychiatrists. And then there is always a stigma attached to seeing a counsellor. The common belief is that only a mentally sick person seeks the help of a counsellor or a psychiatrist. This is a myth— put in simple words—A psychiatrist is a medial person—a doctor and can handle each and every psychological aspect of personality or psychodynamics. A counsellor only focuses on social roles and a few simple emotional problems. Counselling simply means problem solving by aiding the counsellee to learn the skills of making choice and managing his life's role. Psychiatry is concerned with severe psychological disorders which may even require institutional care. A counsellor deals with less severe disorders which seriously or adversely affect easy adjustment. Therefore a counsellee could be any normal human being, who, for some reason is having difficulty to gather strength to cope and is therefore maladjusted. Let me cite an example:

Ms. X is a perfectly normal lady married for several years with a child. She is intelligent, has a career and is financially comfortable. She was living a comfortable life till one day she felt her world was coming crumbling down because her husband was seeing another woman. 'X' tried everything within her power to save her marriage—she cried, begged, pleaded, fought, nagged—but unfortunately these were all negative approaches. These were only pushing him away more towards the other woman. She was devastated and desperate, finally she consulted a counsellor. 'X' came regularly and had intensive counselling meetings—through which she learnt to look at her problem with an analytical mind. The 'Counsellor' helped her to gather all her positive strengths to deal with the situation. She realized that thought the termination or continuation of the relationship between her husband and his friend was not within her control; she definitely had the power to make her life more constructive, more meaningful and then the decision whether she wanted to continue in the marriage or not was quite within her power.

That did the magic! She decided, to stay on, but at the same time started emphasizing on her career, her health, her child and in total on herself as an individual. She stopped feeling helpless and told the counsellor that she now felt strong enough to cope with the situation in a better and positive manner. She is a happier person now and believes strongly that her husbands relationship is just a phase which will wear out with time. Even if it does not she feels she will be able to handle it in a more rational and matured manner. In case Ms. X had decided to walk out of her marriage it would be purely her decision— the 'C's role was to give her an insight into each and every aspect of all the probabilities. Had she continued with her bitterness and anger, she could have turned into a severely maladjusted person which would have affected her home and most importantly her child.

Another case was that of an adolescent girl'S' who was suffering from enuresis or bed-wetting. A few interviews with her revealed to the 'C' that 'S' harbours a special attachment for her father. Unfortunately for 'S' the father is an introvert and aloof person. The father, however, was completely unaware about 'S's feelings. It is a typical family where each member just does his bit, has compartmentalized role and hardly interacts. However the 'C' felt that each member also cared for one another deeply and had the best intentions for each other. They did not know how to communicate their feelings. A few family therapy sessions were arranged where the 'C' helped the members to communicate their feelings in the simplest manner possible, for example, 'S' said to her father 'Daddy I want to buy a gift for you on your birthday'. The father said a simple 'thank you' with the help of 'C' he also told 'S' that he really loves her and cares for her. 'S' and her family members continue to see the 'C' at regular intervals. Their interaction with each other seems to have become easier and more fluid. But the wonderful result of this all was that 'S' has got rid of her bed-wetting problem, of course, this also involved quite a few bed time rules and other disciplines but 80 per cent of the credit goes to the fact that a comfortable and happy father-daughter relationship could be established.

Counselling is available in all leading schools in Delhi and other cities in India. Family counselling can be sought at several voluntary organisations like Sanjeevani at Defence Colony in Delhi; at Sampark in G.M. Modi Hospital, Press Enclave, Saket, Delhi; at

Samvedana, 'S' Block, G.K. II, Delhi and most leading hospitals. But a counsellee should take a lot of care to find a qualified and good counsellor.

In conclusion, I would like to say that the mental equilibrium of a person or a family system tolerates a limited number of traumatic events, according to their importance and nature. But if these unhealthy factors produce pressures beyond tolerable limits, mental and emotional symptoms appear. If such pressures, continue, these symptoms may become critical and serious. An individual and family both constitute a biosocial system. Both can be healthy or unhealthy depending on their capacity to appreciate environmental realities and to fight them forcefully and effectively. Counselling just helps a person to recognize that force and effectivity within him. So if and when needed, do not shy away from counselling; make the best use of it before it becomes too late.

70

PATHOLOGY

Dr. Abhilasha Chaturvedi

In modern medicine, clinical examination is being supported by appropriate lab investigation and imaging techniques, etc., to confirm the provisional diagnosis made by the pathologist and thus pinpointing the treatment accurately.

Broadly, lab investigations can be grouped as routine investigation and specific investigation.

Routine Blood Test

(1) Haemoglobin

This estimation gives information about the red blood pigment in the blood, thus indirectly giving the information, about oxygen carrying capacity of the person. Ideal haemoglobin level is 14 gm per cent approx. But Indian female population is generally having 10-12 gm per cent haemoglobin. Persons having less than 11 gm per cent haemoglobin are considered to be Anaemic.

Particularly in Indian rural population we can see the haemoglobin level going down up to 2-3 gm per cent during pregnancy. In these cases delivery is very risky in spite of having best treatment facilities.

(2) TLC

This is the number of white blood cells present in the blood. The normal range is 5000-10000 cells/cu mm of the level. The count rises during acute bacterial infections and goes down during viral infection and typhoid, etc.

(3) DLC

This is the estimation of percentage of various types of white blood cells, viz., Polymorphism, Lymphocytes, Eosinophils, Monocytes and Basophils.

(4) ESR

This investigation gives information about the level of gamaglobulins in the blood. ESR rises beyond 20 mm in first hour. It also shows presence of various chronic diseases like Tuberculosis and presence of various cancers in the body. ESR should always be done when acute phase of disease is over, otherwise the values may be misleading.

(5) Blood Group and Rh

There are four types of blood groups viz. A, B, O, and AB and any of them can be Rh positive or Rh negative.

Although the range of Rh negative population is less than 15 per cent Rh negative woman if married to Rh positive man, carries a high risk of having complications during delivery for the mother and child both.

As a general rule, every human being should know his or her blood group with certainty.

(6) Routine Urine Examination

Routine urine examination is for the presence of albumin and sugar. Microscopic examination is done for the presence of pus cells and particulate matter like casts which gives important information indicating kidney diseases. Presence of pus cells indicates urinary infections. Glucose is present in the urine of diabetic patients.

Routine investigations are not very costly and should be done during pregnancy, before surgery, during fever, etc.

Testing for the malarial parasite in the blood film is very important and done routinely in the epidermis of malaria.

Blood Sugar measurement is very frequently done in potential diabetics and in pregnant and pre-operative patients as a part of routine. This is done in fasting stage and at the heavy dose of glucose or meal. (2 Hr. post prandial) In strongly suspected cases full glucose tolerance test (GTT) is done.

There are other specific investigations like lipid profile, liner profile, Torch profile, hormone profile and many other types of blood tests. They are done on the advise of specialists.

There is another branch of pathology which deals with the study of bacterial infections by doing their culture sensitivity in various body fluids.

Other lab investigations are cytology and histopathology in which we examine various scrapings for the presence of malignant cells and various biopsy material are tested in detail.

Some other common special investigations, which are very frequently done in gynae clinics, are Urine Test for pregnancy. These are done very fast. They do not require very highly specialized laboratories and can be done by the patients themselves at their homes. Many companies are marketing this type of test kits. These kits are very sensitive and can diagnose the presence of pregnancy even when the patient has just missed 2-3 days of her menses. They are freely available in market.

Other home kits are for the presence of detecting certain types of hormones like L.H. Surge. By detecting L.H. Surge, ovulation can be pinpointed and timing of intercourse can be planned in order to achieve or avoid pregnancy.

Home blood sugar and urine sugar measurement strips are very useful in monitoring of diabetic patients. These are also quite simple and economical.

In modern era no topic is complete without mentioning AIDS. AIDS detection is easily done in almost all pathology labs and blood banks. It is very important for the public to know that there is a window period of approx. 90 days between the exposure to infection and the test becoming positive. In highly suspected cases the test should be repeated after a period of three months. The Elisa Positive are submitted to a very sophisticated western Blot Technique for the confirmation of the diagnosis.

Vaginal cytology for the detection of malignant cells is a routine investigation in almost all developing countries. All the women of child bearing age should go for annual PAP smear test. In this the vaginal scrapings are taken and sent for predicting the cancer of cervix. Routine PAP smear is a very relevant examination in our country because of very high incidence of carcinoma of cervix in India. This is a painless test and cost effective for the mass screening of general population and can be done everywhere easily. The only point is awareness among patients, paramedical staff and policy makers. By picking up early cases of pre-cancerous lesions the disease can be prevented and cured completely. In India the carcinoma of cervix is the commonest cancer among women of childbearing age. That is why it is very essential to have this type of mass screening programms.

Similarly breast cancer can also be detected early by doing fine needle aspiration cytology, (FNAC) of suspicious masses. Generally in cancer prevention awareness and early diagnosis is key to the problem and cytology is the most important tool for fighting the disease.

71

INFECTIOUS VIRAL DISEASES

Dr. Manjula Verma, M.S.

Measles

An acute infectious disease of childhood caused by a specific virus (micro-organism). The earliest description of measles was given by the noted Arab physician Abu Bact (865-925). Causitive virus was isolated by Enders and his colleagues in USA. In 1958, measles vaccine was first used in USA and in 1963, vaccine was licensed for use in clinical trials.

Measles is endemic virtually in all parts of the world. It tends to occur in epidemic when the proportion of susceptible children reaches about 40 per cent.

In India, measles is a major cause of disability and a significant contributor to childhood deaths. Prior to immunization programme, cyclical increase in the incidence of measles were recorded every third year. Death rate in hospitalized cases was 4 per cent with a range of 1.8 per cent to 7.6 per cent. Statistical data shows that the death rate in developing countries is 2-15 per cent as compared to 0.2/10,000 notified cases in developed world. Thus, measles is still a leading killer (1 million of 42 million infected children) among vaccine preventable diseases of childhood.

The only source of infection is a case of measles. Secretions of the nose, throat and upper respiratory tract of a case of measles during the prodromal period of pre-eruptive stages of rush are the infective material. Measles is highly infectious during prodromal period and at the time of infection. The period of communicability is approximately 4 days before and 5 days after the appearance of the rashes.

Characteristics

Measles effects virtually everyone in infancy or childhood, but no age is immune if there was no previous immunity status. It tends to be severe in malnourished children, population density (crowding) and movement especially during winter tend to result in epidemics.

Transmission occurs directly from person to person by droplet infections and portal of entry is respiratory tract. Incubation (lag period) is commonly 10 days and 14 days to appearance of rashes.

There are three stages in the natural history of measles; viz; prodromal or pre-eruptive (rash) stage, eruptive (rash) stage and post-eruptive (rash) stage.

It is characterised by fever, cold with sneezing and nasal discharge, cough, redness of the eyes, lacrimation occasionally there may be vomiting or diarrhoea. A day or two before appearance of rashes typical spots pin-head bluish white (Koplik's) appear in mouth opposite first and second molars. These spots are diagnostic of measles infection.

Rashes are typical dusky red flot or raised beginning behind the ears and spread rapidly in a few hours over face and neck and then extend down the body taking 2 to 3 days.

Post-rash stage the child is weak and susceptible to other bacterial or viral infections.

Measles may be associated with serious infections like pneumonia, other respiratory tract infections and infection of ear. The most serious is the infection of brain (Encephalitis).

No treatment is available till now. Measles is best prevented by active immunization. The most effective time for vaccination is 9 months.

Eradication of measles can be achieved by isolation, achieving immunization rates of 95 per cent and ongoing vaccination against measles through successive generation of children.

Chicken-Pox

Chicken-pox is an acute, highly infectious disease caused by a virus. It is worldwide in distribution and occurs in both epidemic and endemic forms.

Chicken-pox occurs primarily among children under 10 years of age. Few escape infection until adulthood. One attack gives durable protection. Infection during pregnancy carries a risk for the foetus and the neonate chicken-pox shows a seasonal trend in India, the disease occuring mostly during the first six months of the year. Over crowding favours transmission.

Chicken-pox is transmitted from person to person by droplet infection. Many can be infected by direct contact. The virus enters the body through upper respiratory tract.

The lag period (incubation) is usually 14 to 16 days, although extents as wide as 7-21 days have been reported. The clinical cause of chicken-pox can be divided into two stages, i.e., pro-eruptive stage and eruptive stage.

Onset is sudden with mild or moderate fever, pain in back, shivering and malaise lasting for 24 hours when the rashes start coming. Rashes may be the first sign in children. The distinctive features of the rashes are—central distribution, i.e., abundant rashes appear first on trunk and then come on face, arms and legs where they are less abundant. The rashes may noted as clear fluid filled eruptions ("dew drops" on the skin). The fever usually not high but has exacerbations.

In most cases it is mild and self-limiting disease and death rate is less than 1 per cent in uncomplicated cases. The most sensitive means of diagnosis is examination of fluid filled eruptions and their typical central distribution.

There is no specific treatment for chicken-pox. The usual control measures are isolation, disinfection of articles soiled with secretions.

Precaution is the only measure available to fight against this disease.

No serious attempts were made in the past as it was not considered a health priority. A live attenuated vaccine from Japan is extensively studied in field trials. However, opinion is divided about need for a vaccine against chicken-pox as it may be disastrous, if it is postponed from childhood, when it is mild, to adulthood where it is more severe.

It is caused by a virus, it is primarily a childhood disease of worldwide prevalence in urban communities most adults would have had chicken-pox. Transmission is via airborne inhalation if respiratory section from chicken-pox patient or by direct contact with skin lesions and the immunity is life long.

Adults may have malaise and fever for 1 or 2 days' prodromal period is absent in children. There is a rash which rapidly progresses from vesicular to ousting stages over a period of 3-4 days. Crusts separate after about one week leaving a shallowpit which soon disappears. Rash is profuse on the head and trunk and on areas of irritation rash is profuse in adults.

The patient is from 1-2 days before appearance of the rash to 5 days after.

Complications secondary skin sepsin.

Pneumonitis particularly in pregnant woman. Chicken-pox in pregnancy foetal malformation may occur particularly during first trimester-low-birth weight, short limbs, eye, brain damage. Newborn up to 4 weeks after birth may develope severe disease if the mother has rash within 7 days of birth or when contact is post-natal and mother is non-immune. Diagnosis is very simple after rash has appeared.

Prevention

It is customary to exclude children from school until the rash has resolved, but the usefulness of this practice is questionable as most children will develope illness eventually. Patient should be isolated. Varicellar sorter immunoglobin should be given. Susceptible immune suppressed patient. Pregnant women, newborn prone to develope severe disease and complication.

Small-Pox

During nineteenth century, small-pox played havoc causing death and disability like blendness, etc., not only in India but also all over the world. Fourth king of France died of small-pox. It was a dreaded disease worse than the modern AIDS.

Thanks to small-pox vaccination. Small-pox has been eradicated from the world, though like plague it can return with a vengeance story of vaccine preparation is interesting.

Kundalini

The complete realization of 'Brahm' can be achieved by means of the six *chakras* in their proper order. The practice of psyco-physiological techniques will lead towards better health and realization of inner solid strength.

We have evolved from primarily physically motivated animal to a mentally motivated animal and as a result we have lost a lot of our physical strength and capacity to endurance. It could be that the strength and endurance of our cave dwelling ancestors still lies locked within our Central Nervous System (namely brain and spinal cord). This latent energy is called "Kundalini" and is symbolized by a snake coiled three and a half times. The symbology by a snake gives us the secret implications of Kundalini. The snake, symbolizing the procreative urge, symbolizes wisdom as well.

If such an energy as Kundalini does exist, it may be released only through the mind exerting careful stimulation at the point where Kundalini is most apt to manifest.

Snakes as shown are always coiled. This coiling of snake is preparation for striking out and it is in just such a manner that Kundalini lies within us compressed like a spring, ready to change from potential static energy into kinetic manifestations under proper conditions. The three coil represents three states of energy—positive, negative and neutral, while half coil represent Kundalini as always on the verge of changing from static to kinetic manifestations.

The awakening of Kundalini is done through "Laya Yoga".

72

ENDOSCOPY

Dr. Vandana Bansal

During the past few years enormous progress has been made in the field of endoscopic surgery, not only in gynaecology but also in many other surgical disciplines.

Most traditionally procedures performed by laparotomy can now be performed by a minimally invasive technique.

Surgeons today prefer operating under endoscopic vision. The endoscopy is composed of extremely thin threads of bendable glass, which transmits light and images back to the viewer. The doctor can looking through the endoscope, make a diagnosis. By inserting special instruments, the physician or doctor or gynaecologist can also take specimens or remove foreign objects.

The fibre optics technology combined with the latest in micro surgical instruments makes laproscopy one of the most versatile tools available to gynaecologists. The Laproscopy helps to find out the cause of pelvic pain, identity tissue abnormalities and evaluate fertility. During laproscopy, some types of abnormal tissue growths may be removed from organs.

A clear view of the inside are the benefits of laproscopy, an outpatient diagnostic procedure. Doctors uses a long slender, telescope like instrument to view ovaries, fallopian tubes and uterus. The laparoscope contains thin fibre of glass that shine light inside body and series of magnifying lenses are used for viewing. After it is inserted through a small incision the laparoscope can be turned in any direction, so doctors can see pelvic organs from many angles.

Hysteroscopy is a procedure that allows a view directly inside uterus. Hysteroscopy done without incision. It helps the doctor to identify the cause of uterine problems.

Hysteroscopy is commonly done to determine the cause of usually heavy or long periods, bleeding between periods, or post menopausal bleeding. In certain situations, it may be done to evaluate the cause of severe menstrual cramps.

Also Hysteroscopy may sometimes be used to check for cause of infertility or the inability to carry pregnancies to term.

Hysteroscopy is used in two ways. To look inside the uterus for problems such as abnormal growths. Diagnostic Hysteroscopy done. If growths or other problems are found, doctor may remove them during operative Hysteroscopy. After dilation of the cervix the Hysteroscope is inserted through the cervical canal to visualize the important landmarks within the uterine cavities.

During the past few years enormous progress has been made in the field of Endoscopic surgery in Gynaecology.

Operative Laparoscopy is today replacing conventional Gynaecological surgery. 70 per cent of Gynaecological surgery is done Laparoscopy.

Major Gynaecological surgeries are being tackled Laparoscopically.

Advantages

The advantages of operative Laparoscopy are governed by the three basic principles of all surgery, viz., surgical gentleness and elegance efficacy and effectiveness.

There is minimal tissue trauma, resulting in rapid return of treated organs to normal physiology. It is a minimally invasive surgery, adhering to the principles of micro surgery. There is no drying of the tissue as it is a closed surgical procedure. Pneumoperitoneum and tendelenberg position pack away intestines gently and give an excellent exposure of pelvic organs, magnification allows the lesions to be identified and accurately treated, gently and delicate instruments without any damage to the surrounding tissues.

Efficiency

Operative Laparoscopy results, in terms of excision of pathology, functional recovery and pregnancy rates are some.

Cost Effectiveness

Laparoscopic surgery has the advantage of short hospitalisation, minimal post-operative discomfort and restrictions and early return to work. Operative Laparoscopy promotes a totally new therapeutic approach in which diagnosis, therapy and prognosis are achieved simultaneously instead of consecutively.

Indications

Basic

(1) Tubal sterilization

(2) Biopsies

(3) Coagulation of mild endometriosis

(4) Aspiration of small ovarian cysts

Intermediate

(1) Lysis of mild to moderate adhesions

(2) Coagulation of moderate endometriosis

(3) Exploration of small ovarian cysts

(4) Uterine suspension

(5) Salpingectomy and for Ectopic

(6) Removal of weak clips for reversal of tubal sterilization

(7) Treatment of tortured adnexae

(8) Endoscopic Ligatures

(9) Chemical Hemostasis

(10) Lasers

(11) Stapling devices\endoclips

(12) Insufflators

(13) Electronic CO_2 pneumo insufflators

(14) Air pneumo insufflators

(15) Irrigation suction apparatus

(16) Light source

(17) Light cable

(18) Video camera

(19) Sterile cloth bad for accessory instruments.

Hysteroscopy

Indications

(1) Directed biopsies
(2) Cannulation of blocked ostia
(3) Removal of intrauterine foreign bodies
(4) Removal of endometrial polyps
(5) Lysis of intrauterine adhesions
(6) Division of uterine septa
(7) Removal of sub mucous myoma
(8) Ablation of Endometrium (TCRE)
(9) Hysteroscopic sterilization

Armamentarium

(1) Hysteroscopes
  (a) Panoramic
  (b) Contact
  (c) Microcolpo Hysteroscope
(2) Light source and cable
(3) Accessory instruments for operative Hysteroscopy.

Extensive

(1) Cuff salpingostomy
(2) Salpingostomy for ectopic pregnancy
(3) Lysis of extensive adhesions
(4) Excision of moderate to severe endometriosis
(5) Enucleation of ovarian cysts (Endometriotic dermoid)
(6) Cophorectomy
(7) Myomectomy
(8) Tubal anastomosis
(9) Hysteregtomy
(10) Pelvic aortic Lymphadenectomy
(11) Suspension operations for prolapse, stress incontinence

Operations on the tube : Total

Operations on the ovary conservative : Total

Operation on Adnexa

Operations for Endometriosis

Operations on the uterus

Operations for assisted reproduction techniques

Adhesiolysis Pelvic, Lysis of mild, moderate severe adhesions

Armamentarium required for Laparoscopy operation.

(a) Telescope
(b) Tracer cannula
(c) Grasping forceps
(d) Scissors
(e) Section irrigation apparatus
(f) Morcellators
(g) Monopolar electro coagulation
(h) Bipolar electro coagulation
(i) Endo coagulation
(j) Resectoscopes
(k) Lasers
(l) Video camera

There are several substantial advantages of operative hysterscopy to the patient, surgeon and hospital.

(1) Short hospital stay
(2) No incision
(3) Minimal post-operative pain
(4) Rapid recovery and early resumption of full activities
(5) Lower costs
(6) Surgery performed more expeditiously and exactly.

73

MASSAGE

Dr. Vatsala Samant

In India massage has been practised since ancient times. There are many forms of massage styles may differ but all show the common intension of mobilising the natural healing properties of the body in order to help maintain or restore optimal health. A variety of gliding, kneeding and percussive strokes are used along with deep circular movements and vibrations in order to relax muscles, improve circulation and increase mobility.

Nowadays doctors hiring massage therapists to work with patients receiving from a with range of conditions such as joint injuries, chronic backache, neck pain, arthritis sciatica, headache, etc.

How does massage works? When muscles are chronically tense or over worked waste products such as lactic acid accumulates in the muscles. Lactic acid causes soleness, stiffness and even muscle spasm. Massage improves circulation in and out of the muscles and helps elimination of lactic acid a waste product and it eases discomfort. Increase if blood flow brings fresh fuel and oxygen to the body tissues which improves the healing process after the injury and speed recuperation from disease. Hippocrates father of western medicine, in the 5th century wrote about benefits of rubbling better known as massage, it can bind a joint that is two loose and loosen a joint that is too rigid. Massage has long been known to have a great many beneficial effects, physical as well as mental, massage is now recognised for its healing and relaxing potentials, sleeping is improved, one feels more energetic there are is an over all sense of well being.

A proper massage is generally safe for most people, but a massage improperly performed on someone who has suffered an injury or illness can cause damage.

Massage should be avoided when any of these conditions are present, fever, acute inflamation or infection, malignancy jaundice, varicose veins, burns, etc.

In India from time memorial there is a custom of massaging after delivery by barbeis wife. Quite often due to ignorance and immediate use of massage after delivery has resulted in phlerits of white leg an inflamatory condition of the legs giving rise to swelling and pain.

Massage after delivery should be started after about 15 days after normal delivery and one month after operative delivery if there are no complication of child birth and to begin with it should be mild with oil application before bath.

74

HOMEOPATHY

Dr. Vatsala Samant

Homeopathy is a Greek word meaning seekness. Homeopathy began in early 19th century. Dr. Samuel Hahnemann a German physician was disiller seemed with excess of allopathic medicines. He had trust in healing powers of exercise, fresh air, and nourishing diet. However he was not satisfied with the results of these measures and started exploring other means of treatment. He began to test some common medicines on himself, the first medium being cinchona (source of natural quinine which was used to treat malaria, despite the fact that he was healthy on taking cinchona, he developed fever with chills, thirst, and headache, i.e., symptoms of malaria. Hahnemann decided that the effectiveness of the drug in the treatment of malaria came from its ability to cause symptoms to those of the diseases, i.e., like cures like, i.e., a substance that produces certain symptoms in a healthy person can cure seek person who shows the same symptoms.

He used minute doses to avoid side effects caused by large amount of doses.

There was a rapid spread of Homeopathic treatment in the 19th century.

Homeopaths believe that illness is not localised in one organ but instead involves the entire person body and minds they treat the whole person body and mind. They see symptoms as positive sign that the body try to defend itself against the underlying disease. In fact, homeopathic drugs may sometimes temporarily aggravate symptoms as they stimulate the bodys' self-healing mechanism.

Most of the homeopathic remedies are derived from various plants, minerals, animal or chemical sources such as marigold flowers, onions, calcium carbonate, extracts from honeybee.

Homeopathic therapy is being recommended in treatment of chronic diseases lile allergies, headaches, arthritis, cotitis, peptic ulcer, high blood pressure, obesity, anaemia and hormonal imbalance.

75

WATER OR HYDROTHERAPY

Dr. Vatsala Samant

The idea of using water to cure illness and preserve health is as old as civilization. Relationship of water is to cleanliness, relaxation and health. Water from spas have medicinal properties seeking cure for everything from Acne to anxiety, airing water of varying temperature and pressure is recognised as an effective course of treatment for a variety of health problems. Heat dilates blood vessels increasing the circulations a hot feet bath helps uncloging congested nasal passages reducing swelling and allowing more air to pass. Heat also relaxes muscles eases stiffness of joints and relieves aches and pains. This treatment is contra indicated on infants, aged and during pregnancy cold causes blood vessels to contract, reducing blood flow swelling and conflamation and also fever and cold packs are effective in the treatment of headache, nose bleeds, muscle spasms, bruises and splains. If one likes a hot water baths and then a cold water bath blood vessels first dilate then contract improving blood circulation and this relieves muscular cramps, reduces inflamation of tissues and helps the body to fight infecting and heal more quickly. Siby bath is used to treat abdominal ailmants and injuries. For relaxation water bath should be tepid baths beyond cleanliness have soothing effect on mind and body water can act as cushion for baby during pregnancy and it is comfortable for them to exercise in water, when exercise is needed to pregnant women and can prepare them for the physical demands of childbirth exertion required of the heart and lungs is a good aerobic activity. Swimming is very popular but now water exercises of all kinds are becoming increasingly popular for everyone.

76

AYURVEDA'S THERAPY OR MEDICINE

Dr. Vatsala Samant

Ayurveda means science of life or longevity, Ayurvedic medicine is 2500 years or more old and it is considered the first organised approach to health based on natural phenomena and not on magic superstition and spiritual forces. Illness developes as a result of external dishormoney. The body's innate ability to heal itself provides the unifying force behind Ayurvedic medicine which also emphasis is on teaching preventive health care so that one can enjoy longer and healthier life.

We fail to take advantage of our own healing powers and the effect of which is to become sick. Stressful lifestyles of modern life, insuitable diet (junk diets), engaging in activities out of tune with the seasons can upset the delicate balance required necessary for health through infectious diseases can be disruptive. When we are in balance with ourselves and our environment we are far less likely to succumb to ailments of any kind.

According to Ayurveda, the critical balance of the body depends on three basic life forces or doshas which are thought of as fundamental elements underlying human functionary. The three doshas are Vat, Pitta, Kapha.

1. Vat meas air which is supposed to produce movements.

2. Pitta fire dosha means heat dihydration, digestion, serving as a transformative interforce between Vat and Kapha. It is the one that converts material substances Vatic gaseous.

3. Kapha allied to earth, which is a stabilising force that is responsible for bodily structure. According to Ayurveda, each of us is born with a unique ratio of these three Doshas though one can predominate, the basic constitution in body type, temperament and also the kind of chronic disorders to which one is most susceptible,

Pitta types tend to be passionate, argumentative and quick to anger and can suffer from rashes, heart throb and peptic ulcer.

The doshas characterize the world around us foods, seasons, time of the day, they suggest a diet, daily routine and activities that will help each one maintain balance, for example, in spring a kapha season predominantly. Kaph type will probably advised to go light on Kaph aggravating tools us heavy dairy products, otherwise body will be forced to divest itself of the excess of Kaph or mucous a spring cold foods and herbs may subdue or increase doshas, for example, pungent chillies increase pitta, while sweets or stardy foods cause welling up of Kaph.

When illness strikes a person despite taking necessary precautions, Ayurvedic medicine offers an arsenal of cures, many herbal proteins and even surgery. Research has shown evidence of minor and major surgery, cosmetic, skin grafting, removal of gall-bladder during the prehistoric period as shown by the Indian scriptures written thousands of years ago.

There are two types of Ayurvedic medicines, one is practised by Ayurvedic doctors for those who ills, the other is practised by each and every person as a way of staying healthy, when a person observes, any disturbances of three doshas appropriate adjustments are made in diet, exercise and patterns of thought and emotions to bring the balance in the dosha and illness is elegantly sidestepped. Now even the W.H.O. has recognised Ayurvedic medicines side by side with Allopathic medicines.

Ayurvedic medicine deals in an integrated way with body and mind, any disturbance of the three doshas will be reflected on both mental and physical levels, for example, a disturbance of value produces numbness and pain (Physically) and anxiety (Mentally). A mental event such as worry or fasting (Physical can aggravate Vatal). There was a time when Ayurveda and yoga were distinct, nowadays the trend is bringing the two together.

Ayurvedic treatment consists of adjusting diet to suit ones constitution and the season of the year and elaborate herbal medicines others employ spices and turmeric to dry up phlogm.

To cleanse the body of accumulated wastes Ayurveda has developed several procedures known as Panchkarma these include herbal steam treatment, oil massage, nasal purging, and the use of laxatives and medicated enemas but one has to consult an Ayurvedic practitioners.

77

SCIENCE OF RELAXATION

Dr. Vatsala Samant

Scientist define stress, that it is not only simply an event outside ourselves, but our way of reacting to it and stress is not imposed on us from outside and the cause of stress is known as stress or which may as a natural disaster, war or internal such as feeling of anger or anxiety. It may be physical injury, economic or emotional. The effect of stress produces muscle fatigue, headache, ulcers, asthma, backache, digestive disorders, high blood pressure. Whether the stress comes from a overload of major stressors on a chronic over-reaction to relatively minor ones its immediate is the same rapid pulse, sweating palms, nausea and tension and the physiological reactions are "fight or flight" response which was evolved in animals and human beings living to the wild which helped them to cope with emergency. This response was vital to our anestors to save themselves from a marauding tiger or falling tree, even today it helps us to dodge a speeding car.

Managing stress with relaxation. Just as we have an innate stress response we have the ability to relax and gain control over the stress.

Through relaxation we may not be able to stress-proof life. We can stress guard our body and mind.

Simple relaxation aids are helpful, relaxing with a hobby, or exercise, listening to be music, knitting etc. Shavasan corpse pose is very useful to relax.

The workplace can be a major source of stress and physical tension. These are methods of relaxation which can diffuse stress without leaving your desk.

78

TIPS FOR MEDITATION AND ALSO RELAXATIONS

Dr. Vatsala Samant

1. *Isolated environment.* Eliminate. as many distractions as you can.

2. *Focus attention.* Concentrate on a word, picture or sound repeated either silently or aloud.

3. *Passive Attitude.* Don't try to make it happen.

4. *Comfortable position.* Free yourself of tension, wear loose clothing.

5. *Regular practice.*

6. *Formal Position.* A comfortable erect setting position that keeps you relaxed and yet alert.

Meditation

Many people troubled by the stress of modern life. Have turned up to age-old methods of meditation to help them cope with anxiety.

Meditation is a mental exercise aimed at training the mind itself. It emphasizes technique of mental control a happy stillness of mind (William Wordsworth). How this mechanism produces the changes is not known but it certainly relieves stress and eases tension.

It has been observed that meditation lowers oxygen consumption and heart rate and blood pressure. Psychotherapists now use meditation to help patients deal with emotionally changed users. There are two ways, either focussing on an object or to attempt to empty the mind if one chooses a meditation programme at least 20 minutes a day are recommended.

Maharshi Mahesh Yogi started transcendental meditation (TM). TM is easy to learn. Its central feature is the chanting of a secret mantra a single syllable word such as "OM".

EPILOGUE

Dr. Vatsala Samant

An idea of writing a booklet on health for women was there right from the beginning of my medical superintendantship of Kamala Nehru Hospital. But due to workload, illness home problems, I was unable to put at the on paper.

After my retirement from Nazreth hospital in 1995 the seed of writing was sown. Not being a writer it took me some time to sit down and put on paper my ideas about health awareness on paper but even then concentration was lacking. A small book was ready after reading and writing but it was impossible to publish it due various factors. When I got a publisher they wanted some more chapters to be added and that took more time to complete the book.

Even if one woman in ten benefits by reading this book on health awareness one I shall be have my dream come true.

What I am today is due the women of Allahabad who had trust in me regarding ailments and nothing acts to a doctor better than the trust or confidance in you, which is just like a shot of adranal in worth a million dollars.

I thought it would be in the fitness of thing to dedicate this book to women of Allahabad. And so this book is a culmination of a long dream which had begun long ago.

Index

Abdominal
    Muscles, Exercises for the, 44
    T.B., 118
Abnormalities, 35
Abortion, 53, 132
    Criminal, 53
    Habitual, 53
    Repeated, 77
    Symptoms, 53
    Therapeutic, 54
Acupuncture, 196, 219
    points, 196
Aerobics, 203
    Action Plan; 203
    Advantage, 203
Ageing, 107, 202
AIDS, 61, 179, 181, 183-84
Alzheimers, Systems, 108
Amenorrhoea, 28
Amitrypheline, 237
Anaemia and High Blood Pressure, 48
    Causes of, 243-44
    Diagnosis, 243
    in Pregnancy, 245
    Management, 244
    Treatment, 244
    Worm Infestation, 244
Anannechaphaly Hydrocephalus, 101
Anencephaly, 97
Antenatal
    Care, 47-48, 66
    check-ups, 66
Armamentarium, 277
Artificial Insemination, 81
Aspirin, Do not use, 93
Ayurveda Therapy, 285
Ayurvedic
    medicine, 285-86
    practitioners, 286
ATZ, 181

Babies, Premature, 87
Baby, Sex of the, 51
Backache, 221-22
Backpain, 64
Barrier Methods, 72
Benign Ovarian Tumour, 151
Bleeding, 132
    Irregular, 139
Blood
    Sugar Measurement, 264
    Test, Routine, 263
Breast, 35, 64
    and Nipples, Accessory, 36
    and salivary gland, 187
    are set in action, 49
    Asymmetrical, 36
    Cancer Early Detection, 173
    Cancer, Transplant Therapy for, 173
    Disease, When to suspect, 173
    Feeding, 89
    Lump in the, 157
    pendulous, 36

Caessarian Section, 135
Calcium
    Content of food, 124
    Foods, 198

Cancers, 69, 163, 169
Breast, 168, 171
Breast, Advice, 172
Breast, Investigations, 172
Breast, Symptoms, 171
Breast Treatment, 172
Causes of, 155
Cervical, 159
detecting tests, 157
of the Ovary, Primary, 161
of the Reproductive Organs, 159
of the Reproductive System, 155-56
of the Uterine Cervix, 168
of the Vagina, 146
Radio therapy in the treatment of, 165
treatment, 157
What is, 155
Carbohydrates, 194
Carcinoma
Cervix, 163, 266
of the Body of the Uterus, 160
Cataract, 113-14
Congenital, 114
Traumatic, 114
Causes, 79
Cell medicated, 176
Cerebrovascular disease, 232
Chicken-Pox, 268-69
in pregnancy foetal malformation, 270
Child
birth, 48
health programme, 61
Childhood Deformities, 97
Children, How to take Temperature, 93
Clitoris, 23
Complete realization of Brahm, 269
Conception, 39
Sign and Symptom, 40
Congested nasal passages, hot feet bath helps, 283
Contact a Doctor, when to, 209
Contact your Doctor, 94
Conclusion, 212
Contraception, 69
Contraceptive
Devices, Intra Uterine, 17
Non-Steroidal, 72
Steroidal, 71
Counselling :
A Therapy, 259
is available in all leading schools in Delhi, 261
made the best use, 262
Counsellor
helped her to gather all her positive strengths, 260
role is mistaken, 260

Defence Systems of the body, 175
Deficiency of Vit. A, 101
Dehydration, 95
signs of, 95
Delivery, caesarean and forceps, 48
Detect Cancer Early, How to, 174
Development, function and disorders, 35
Dhanurasana, 215
Diabetes, 102, 227
Complications of, 232
Diagnosis, 227
insulin dependent, 228
non-insulin dependent, 228
Risks of Inheriting, 228
Types of, 228
Type 1, 288
Type 2, 229-31
What is, 227
Diagnosis
Criteria for, 227
Mistakes in, 228
Dialation and Curettage, 135

Discharge
Pathological, 145
Puberty, 145
Purulent, 145
Vaginal, 145
Dyslenia, 105
Systems, 105
Dysmenorrhoea, 29

EEG, 255
Embryo, Development of the, 43
Endocrine Influences, 102
Endometrical Biopsy, 135
Endometriosis, 30
Endoscopy, 273
Cost Effectiveness, 274
Indication, 275
Surgery, 273-74
vision, 273
Enuresis, 147
Environmental factors, 228
Episiotomy wound, 63
Epilogue, 291
Exercises,
Advantages of, 205
and Diet, 205
during Pregnancy and after Childbirth, 205

Fallopian Tubes, 21
Family
Counselling, 261
Health, 70
health and education, 259
planning, 61, 67, 68
welfare, 61
Fat, 194
Fatigue, 52, 64, 238
Feeding the baby, 83
Females,
Causes in, 80
Tubal Ligation, 73
Fever, 93
Fibre 193
Fibroid, 162
Fibromayalgia in Children, 235-36
Fibromyoma of the Uterus, 151
Fine needle aspiration cytology, 266
Fitness, 193
FM, 236
Foetal anonia, 101
Food rich in Calcium, 198
Fungus or Virus, 150

Galactorrhea, 37
and infertility, 38
Gamma-Ray Beam, 167
Gastroenteritis, 95
Causes of, 995
Genital Hygiene, 143
Genetic factor, 228
German Measles, 48
Glaucoma, 111
General treatment, 112
varieties of, 111
Giardia or Amoebic infections, 95
Gynaecologist for Infertility, 80
Gynaecomastitis, 36
Gynological Disorders, rush to hospital due to, 208

Haematoma, 64
Haemoglobin mass, 243
Hare Lip and Clef, 97
Health Care means Rolling, 128
Healthy Eating, 206
the Natural Way, 127
Heartburn, 51
Hepatitis
B, 251-52
B Symptoms, 251
toxic, 251
Hermophrodite Eunuchs, 223
Hirsuikism, 223-24
HIV, 48, 181, 184
Homeopathy, 281
therapy, 282

Honeymoon Pyelitis, 148
Hormones, 187
  Ovarian, 188
  Replacement Therapy, 33
HRT cyclic oestrogens and progestron, 24
Humoural, 176
Hypertension, 232
Hypogonadotropic genetic etiology, 24
Hypothyroid, 191
Hypothyroidism, 189-90
Hysterectomy, 136
Hysteria, 225
  Symptoms, 225
  Treatment, 225
Hysteroscopy, 273-74
  Armamentarium, 276
  Extensive, 276

Immunization, 85
  is essential, 85
Infection, 149
  of brain Encephalitis, 268
  of Uterus, 149
  of Vulva, 149
Infectious
  Disease, 102
  viral Diseases, 267
Infertility, 75
Injectable, 71
Insomnia, 52, 257
Instructions, 80
Intersex, 223
Intraoperative Radiotherapy and Radiosurgery, 169
Investigations, 80
  to be performed, 232
Ionizing
  radiation, 167
  in treating, 165
Irradiation Exposure, 102

Kamla Nehru Hospital, 25
Kapha, 285-86
Kraurosis of the Vulva, 153
Kundalini, 270-71

Labia
  majoria, 23
  minora, 23
Labour
  Child-birth, 55
  First stage, 55
  is strenuous, 217
  Pain in, 56
  Second stage, 55
  Third stage, 55
Laproscopy, 136, 273
  operation, 277
Laprotomy, 273
Laya Yoga, 271
Lens in the eye, 113
Leukoplakia, 153
Lima Madena, 24
Linear Accelerators, 167
Lipoprotein metabolism, 232
Limphocyles, 176

Malaria, 241
Male Infertility, cause of, 81
  Vasectomy, 73
Malformations, Congenital, 101
Malpresentation, 132
Mammography, What is, 174
Management, 32, 99
Massage, 279
  should be avoided, 280
  work, How does, 279
Mastitis, 37
  Acute, 37
  Chronic, 37
Maternal death, 47
Maternity, Toll of, 65
Measles, 267-68
  Characteristics, 268
Meditation, 289
  a mental exercise, 289

Menopausal or post-menopausal bleeding, 29
Menopause, 31
Artificial, 32
Delayed, 32
Premature, 32
Menorrhaia, 29
Menses, 27
General Disturbance Associated with, 27
Scanty or Absent, 140
Menstrual bleeding, 25
Menstruation, 27
Abnormalities of, 28
cessation of, 31
infrequent, 29
Mental Retardation, 98
Milk,
Hand expressing, 90
Mind Power, Value of, 128
Minerals, 194
Essentials, 195
Miscellaneous Methods, 73
Monglolism, 103
Morning sickness, 132
Mortality, Maternal, 141
Mother after Child-birth, care for, 144
Motherhood, 131
surrogate, 82
MR Prevention, 99

National and Official Policy, 68
Natural Methods, 73
Necessary Elements of diet, 193
Nervous tension, 28
Newborn Baby,
Care of the, 83
Problems in a, 84

Obesity, 253-54
Causes (Etiology) of, 253
Risk related to, 253
Treatment of, 254
Obstetrics, 39
OM, 290
Operations,
Major, 135
Minor, 135
Operative
hysterscopy, 277
Laparoscopy, 274
Procedures in Obstetrics and gynaecology, 135
Organ, External, 23
Orteoarthritis, 121
Osteoporosis, 123-24
Other Problems, 78
Ovarian
Pedicle, 161
secretion, 27
Ovaries, 21
Ovary, 21

Padmasan, 214
Paediatrician Immediately when to go to your, 84
Pathology, 263
Pathological Causes, 28
Pelvic Floor Muscles, Exercises for, 44
peripheral neuropathy, 232
peritourism, 249
Permanent, 71
Methods, 73
Physical and mental ailments, 219
Physiotherapists, 217
Physiotherapy, 121, 217
Piles, 51
Pitta, 285-86
Planned
parenthood, 67
Small family, 69
PMS Syndrome, 25
Post-menopausal
Bleeding, 161
bare loss, 123

Post-Natal,
    care for Puerperium, 49
    period, 217
    period, Hazards, 63
Predisposing Factors, 97
Pregnancy, 39, 47, 65, 68, 76, 212
    and its Hazards, 131
    Diet During, 197
    Ectopic, 40-41, 131
    Extra Uterine, 40
    Problems During, 51
    Toxemia of, 132
Premarital Sex, 79
Presentation, Symptoms and Signs, 230
Prevalence, 231
Prevention of Rubella, 102
Proteins, 194
Pruritis Vulvae, 146, 153
Pseudo, 28
Psychological
    Changes, 31
    factors, 221
Psycosis, 64
Pubertal bleeding, 29
Puberty, 23
    and adolescence, period between, 23
    Delayed, 24
    Precocious or Early, 24
Puerperal sepsis infection, 64
Puerperium, Hazards of, 63
Pulmonary infection, 117

Radiotherapy for cancer cervix, 166
RCH Reproductive Child Health, 61
Relaxation aids, 287
Renal failure, 232
Reproductive
    Organs, Injury to the, 133
    system, Anatomy of, 21
Rhesus factor, 49
Rheumatoid
    Arthritis, 119
    Arthritis, Symptoms, 119
RH
    factor, 49
    negative, 49
    negative blood, 50
    negative mothers, 86
    positive, 49-50
    positive babies, 86
Rhythm Method, 73
Rubella, 102

Sampark, 261
Samvedana, 262
Sanjeevani, 261
Scanty Menses, 28
Science of Relaxation, 287
Self-Examination, Ways to do, 173
Senile Vaginitis, 109
Sex Education, 183
Sexual glands, 21
Sexually Transmitted Diseases, 150
Shavasana, 213
Siddhasana, 213
Sleep : A Divine Gift, 255
    disturbed, 207, 256
Small-pox vaccination, 270
Sonography, 75-76
Spacing Methods, 70
Spina bifida account, 101
S.T.D., 61
Stress, 207
Surgery, Radiotherapy, and Chemotherapy, 162-63
Symptoms, 113

T cell
    Helper, 177
    Killer, 177
    suppresser, 177
    Types, 176
Temporary, 70

Tetanus infects, 48
Thyroid, 189
    hormone, 190
Thyroxane Treatment to give, 189
Tips for
    Meditation, 289
    Relaxations, 289
Treatment, 81, 113
Triple Antigen, 85
Tuberculosis, 117, 247
    Abdominal, 248-49
    Causes, 247
    Environmental Hygiene, 248
    Meningitis, 24
    Prevention, 248
    Reproductive, 249
    Symptoms, 248
    Treatment, 248
Tubectomy, 136
Tumour, 37
    can become malignant, 162
    of the genital Organs, 151

Ultrasound, 75, 137
Urinary Track Disturbance, 14,
Urine,
    Incentinence of, 147
    Retention of, 148
UTI, 148
Uterus, 21

Vaccines recommended, 85
Vagina, 23
Vaginalcytology, 265
Varicose Veins, 117
Vat, 285
Vitamins, 195
    and their role, 197
Vomiting and Diarrhoea,
    Prevention of, 96
    What to do at Home in case of, 96

Water or Hydrotherapy, 283
What to do, 93
WHO, 70, 286
Who should be screened, 229

Yoga, 211
    Hints and cautions taken to practise, 212
Yogasana, 214
Yogi, Maharshi Mahesh, 290
Young girls, Advice to, 82